14-DAY
Anti-Inflammatory
Diet

G

GALVAN!ZED
Media

This book proposes a program of diet and exercise recommendations for the reader to follow. However, you should consult a qualified medical professional (and, if you are pregnant, your ob-gyn) before starting this or any other diet or fitness program. Please seek your doctor's advice before making any decisions that affect your health or extreme changes in your diet, particularly if you suffer from any medical condition or have any symptom that may require treatment. As with any diet or exercise program, if at any time you experience discomfort, stop immediately and consult your physician.

Mention of specific companies, organizations, or authorities in this book does not imply endorsement by the author or publisher, nor does mention of specific companies, organizations, or authorities imply that they endorse this book, its author, or the publisher.

Distributed by Simon & Schuster

ISBN 9781940358291
Ebook ISBN 9781940358376

Printed in the United States of America on acid-free paper.

Design by Andy Turnbull

THE
14-DAY
Anti-Inflammatory
Diet

Heal your gut, prevent disease and slow aging— one bite at a time!

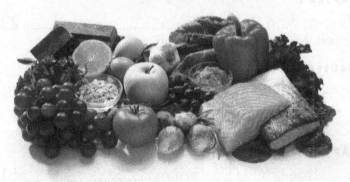

BY MIKE ZIMMERMAN
AND THE EDITORS OF
Eat This, Not That!®

Contents

Why You Need This Book

Learn how chronic inflammation is taking a deadly toll on your body—even right this second—and how you can turn the tide and reclaim your health

THE DRAMATIC STUFF always gets the headlines.

Start at the top: Cancer. So many varieties. So many worthy platforms raising awareness. Even if you've never had it, you know someone who has. How about heart disease? Type 2 diabetes? Stroke? Obesity . . . high blood pressure . . . high cholesterol. . .high blood sugar. Yes, it's like the medical community's Most Unwanted List. They're so popular—meaning unpopular, and hated and feared—because they're so common in our society. They've earned their notoriety.

But there's another silent killer among us (no, not hypertension; something just as dangerous). You don't really know about it because it doesn't get the headlines all those other health issues get. You don't feel it because it just kind of does its nasty thing inside your body at all hours of the day. You go about your business, live your life, and as time goes by, maybe you put on some weight like a lot of people, or a *lot* of weight like a lot of people, maybe your diet isn't as good as it could be like a lot of people's, maybe you spend more time on the sofa as you get older like a lot of people. And through it all, the silent killer does its work. Patient. Persistent. Pernicious.

I first read about chronic inflammation more than 10 years ago when I was a senior editor at *Men's Health* magazine. We did a special report on C-reactive protein, an inflammation marker in the body that could signal an elevated risk for heart disease. At the time, no one had heard about it before. Of all the health issues we covered— and we covered the nastiest—inflammation freaked me out the most. And for all the reasons I just mentioned: It's just in there taking its toll on you *and you never know it*—even if your health markers are otherwise normal. Why is chronic inflammation so scary? I'll get into much more detail in Chapter 1, but the bottled version: It has a hand in virtually every negative health problem you could experience, particularly the Big Ones I just mentioned. This book has the word "diet" in the title, so you may not be surprised to learn that a significant contributor to chronic inflammation comes from what we eat. You may be surprised, however, to find out just which foods trigger it and how many of them are part of your regular menu. Over time, this incessant inflammatory response can lead to weight gain, drowsiness, skin problems, digestive issues, and a host of diseases, from diabetes to obesity to cancer.

To be fair, inflammation has become a bigger part of the overall health and wellness conversation. But it's still in the minor leagues when you talk about media coverage or, in particular, healthcare circles. Example: Your doctor will routinely have conversations about your weight, or blood pressure, or fasting blood sugar/A1C readings. Those are big red flags with easily understood number ranges. But has your doctor ever once mentioned chronic inflammation as a risk factor for your health? I bet not.

Why is that a problem? Well, if you're overweight with blood pressure/blood sugar issues, chronic inflammation has already done a number on you and will continue to do so. But there are a lot of people out there who haven't hit that level yet. You may be, say, moderately overweight with health scores that most doctors would consider "okay," as in no critical red flags at the moment. But your body could be harboring chronic inflammation behind the scenes, *helping, encouraging, pushing* your body toward eventual health issues like type 2 diabetes, inflammation-based diseases, and yes, heart disease and cancer.

That's why, when my friends at *Eat This, Not That!* asked if I'd be interested in helping to create a diet-based book that takes on inflammation, I jumped in. I've been writing and editing health/fitness/weight-loss magazines for millions of people for nearly 20 years. I've co-authored more than a dozen books designed to help people live healthier, more active lives. My mission has always been bringing that positive message to as many people as possible: *You can be healthier.*

Another reason: I see myself in the mirror. I'm not as gray-free as I used to be. I'm a little heavier than I should be. And I don't always eat the way I should. I live in eastern Pennsylvania, which has become ground zero for some of the most amazing craft-brewed East Coast-style IPAs you could ask for. I have a cheese problem. And Pop Tarts and I share a love that dare not speak its name. In short, I'm just as much a candidate for chronic inflammation as anyone. I wanted to learn as much as I could about it so I could do something about it.

There's more. In the last 2 years, I learned more about my family medical history than anyone would want. My father died in 1989 from stomach cancer. Now, stomach or gastric cancer isn't one of the Big Ones that get the headlines. About 26,000 people were diagnosed in 2018 in the U.S., according to the American Cancer Society, and while gastric cancer is more common in places like Japan, 26K doesn't exactly make the disease a hot-button issue. But here's the catch, for me: Stomach cancer is generally an older-person's cancer, with the six out of 10 diagnoses happening after age 65. My father was diagnosed at age 59—and his case was advanced because he'd ignored the symptoms. Still, in my eyes at the time, it wasn't an issue. It was just the thing that killed him. But years later, my father's niece got her stomach cancer diagnosis. She passed away at 53. Then, two years ago, my older sister got her diagnosis. She died in early 2018 at age 55.

So now I'm staring at three close-family stomach cancer fatalities all diagnosed before age 60. And there's that food-stomach relationship thing that I can't avoid. For me, diet now matters more than ever.

So let's talk about this.

As you'll read later on, there are several possible reasons a person can have chronic low-grade inflammation. Some conditions are genetic. But in many cases, especially when you're talking about inflammation from belly fat, or drinking too much, or eating the wrong foods, the cause is pretty obvious. I've interviewed dozens of doctors over the years. Some you've heard of—Mehmet Oz, Travis Stork—and many others you haven't. But with all of them, no matter how extensive we discussed science, research results, how the body works, what-is-or-isn't-healthy, every conversation could be boiled down to one word: *choices.*

Our choices, in many cases, define our health.

That's why the 14-Day Anti-Inflammatory Diet is so exciting. It gives you a chance to take control of your choices for a short period to reverse the cascade of inflammation in your body. Here's a partial list of the benefits:

You'll Attack the Number on the Scale

Yes, we call it a "diet," and yes, it is food-based, so yes, it's designed to help you shed pounds. Here's the thing: Science has shown again and again that certain foods can cause inflammation in the body, while some other foods have anti-inflammatory powers. You'll be leaving the first group behind and embracing the other group. And inflammation is a double-whammy—foods can cause it, but so can toxic fat cells in your body—so you'll be attacking inflammation on both fronts. You'll lower inflammation with food *and* by losing weight.

You'll Attack the Inflammation Damaging Your Body

Inflammation is more than just about weight. By reducing your inflammation levels and eating healthier, you'll reduce and even reverse the damage inflammation inflicts. That means lower risk levels for type 2 diabetes, heart disease, cancer, and a host of other health problems (you'll learn more in chapter 1).

You'll Discover Other Powerful Anti-inflammatory Weapons

Food is a huge inflammation factor—for good or bad—because we eat throughout the day for fuel. So food will be our primary ally. But you'll also learn about some other simple lifestyle changes that also have been scientifically proven to reduce inflammation. You'll fight inflammation on multiple fronts with multiple weapons.

You'll Learn New Ways to Live a Healthier Life

This program lasts 14 days. But it's so easy to continue these good habits for life. After all, inflammation doesn't go away forever just because you adopted a healthier lifestyle for two weeks. It's a lifelong battle, and you'll have all the tools you'll need. Plus, we bet that you'll feel so good after 14 days that you'll simply *want* to continue what you started. All you gotta do is keep going.

Let's begin. Commit to this program for the next 2 weeks and reap the rewards. The journey to a slimmer, healthier body starts now...

CHAPTER

1

Inflammation: Good, Bad, and Very Ugly

How can a natural body process suddenly be so devastating to your health?

W

AIT, WHAT? Inflammation is beneficial and it's *killing* us? What's going on here?

Okay. Take a breath. Let's start at the beginning.

Inflammation is a natural process in the human body. It's an integral part of our immune system's response to an invader. That's it. It's that simple. Examples: You get a cold, your body responds to fight the cold, and you have a spike of inflammation in your body. As that happens, **your body heats up to kill the virus**. Or you cut your finger. Your body

1

mobilizes to heal the cut (notice how the area is temporarily red, swollen, inflamed?). How about an allergic reaction to a bee sting? Scary, if you're not prepared. But that's your body responding to a threat and your immune system goes on the attack.

That's inflammation in a nutshell. In truth, it's an incredibly involved physical process that's loaded with scientific terms you can't pronounce (but we'll try in a moment!). When it's working like it should, it's not just beneficial, but vital to our long-term survival.

So what's the problem? Well, the examples I just gave you are instances of *acute inflammation*, in that they're a temporary response to a threat that heals quickly. A cold goes away in about a week. Ditto to a cut on your finger (unless you really sliced into it). And the allergic response, if treated quickly, recedes over minutes or hours. Acute: It hits, the body responds, the condition heals in a timely and healthy manner. Acute inflammation from that process also dissipates in a timely and healthy manner.

Ah, but sometimes, if conditions in the body are right (meaning really, really wrong), your immune system will keep the body in a constant, long-term state of inflammation—meaning weeks, months, or years—a.k.a. *chronic low-grade inflammation*.

While inflammation is a natural, protective part of the body's immune response, it's only protective in brief doses. When you put your immune system in a state of constant attack, over time, the inflammatory response damages cells. This takes a toll and can cause weight gain, drowsiness, skin problems, digestive issues, and a host of diseases, including diabetes, cancer, and depression.

Over the past few years, researchers have coined

catchy new terms to help describe the inflammation problem. "Metaflammation" describes inflammation from metabolic processes (type 2 diabetes falls under this heading). "Inflammaging" describes how inflammation can accelerate the aging process (gut health, which we'll describe shortly, is a big factor here). No matter how you say it, chronic inflammation is an odd combination of your immune system causing inflammation, attempting to eliminate the perceived threat, and destroying healthy tissue all at the same time. And because it's considered low-grade, most times you have no idea it's even happening. Another silent killer going about its business shortening your life.

In this chapter, we'll reveal all of chronic inflammation's secrets: why it happens, why it hurts us, and what we can do about it. Then we'll talk about how the 14-Day Anti-Inflammatory Diet can be such a powerful weapon against it (which is why we're here, after all). Read on ...

CHRONIC INFLAMMATION: YOUR ANGRY BODY

So the question looms: How can something natural—and designed to be beneficial—be so toxic to our health? Well, it comes down to a simple fact that has been sabotaging humans since the beginning of our time: We have something good and we misuse and abuse it. Now, not *everything* is the human's fault, but here are some of the common causes of chronic inflammation:

An outside infection that's hard to kill: For our purposes here, real but rare.

Hot Zone

A partial list of health conditions linked to chronic inflammation

- Cancer
- Heart disease (atherosclerosis)
- Type 2 diabetes
- Metabolic syndrome
- Obesity
- Visceral (abdominal) fat
- Rheumatoid arthritis
- Chronic obstructive pulmonary disorder (COPD)
- Periodontitis
- Dementia (including Alzheimer's)
- Allergies
- Lupus
- Gastritis
- Pulmonary fibrosis
- Inflammatory bowel diseases (Crohn's disease, colitis)
- Multiple sclerosis
- Chronic fatigue
- HIV
- Celiac disease
- Osteoarthritis
- Cystic fibrosis
- Pelvic inflammatory disease
- Parkinson's disease
- Erectile dysfunction
- Depression
- Asthma

Genetics: Some people inherit health issues. It's not fair, but it's a fact. Some health conditions are a product of chronic inflammation; others cause it. Either way, inflammation is linked to a whole lot of problems.

Environment: Where you live may not be good for you. Millions of people have no control over this—not many have the ability to just pull up stakes and move to another state and/or country. But pollution, water quality, air quality, and a host of other environmental factors can contribute to chronic inflammation.

Lifestyle: This is the one we need to talk about because this is the one we can control the most. This is the "misuse and abuse" part I just mentioned. All of our biggest lifestyle deficiencies are linked to chronic inflammation. Conversely, if you live a healthy lifestyle to reverse those deficiencies, inflammation levels will drop. What are those "deficiencies?" You can probably guess.

- **Unregulated stress**
- **Lack of physical activity**
- **Lousy sleep**
- **Smoking**
- **Alcohol abuse**
- **And, of course, poor diet**

For now, let's talk about the food. Think about it: Certain foods cause an inflammatory response in your body. Your body tries to take care of it, but boom, before your body knows it you've eaten another inflammatory food. Your body—between the stress, lack of exercise, horrible sleep, and constant junk food—can't catch a break.

Signs of Acute Inflammation
(as described 2,000 years ago by Celsus, who wrote a series of Roman encyclopedias)

These symptoms are short-lived.

Rubor = Redness
Tubor = Swelling
Calor = Heat
Dolor = Pain

Signs of Chronic Low-Grade Inflammation
(brought on by poor food and lifestyle choices)

These symptoms stick around. The problem is connecting these symptoms to chronic inflammation itself, as they all appear to be signs of poor lifestyle choices rather than a diagnosable condition. But if you have them, chances are you have inflammation issues, as well.

- **Weight gain**
- **Fatigue**
- **Skin problems (acne, dermatitis, rosacea)**
- **Digestive issues**

Of course, by "poor diet," we're talking about the typical American diet, which is full of inflammation-inducing foods. Chapter 3 will go into far more detail, but think fried foods, refined flours and sugars, hormone- and antibiotic-laden animal products, synthetic sweeteners, and artificial food additives. So, if you're constantly noshing on these items, your body will begin to transition into a state of chronic inflammation. This inflammatory, high-energy (read: sugary and starchy) diet builds belly fat, reduces levels of gut-healthy probiotics, induces weight gain, causes joint

Thank You for Not Smoking

This can't be surprising news, but if you smoke, you're inflaming your entire body every time you light up. A 2016 study in the *Journal of Leukocyte Biology* noted the discovery of why smoking causes such an inflammatory response in the body. It's not the smoke. It's not the chemicals. It's not the tar. Apparently, the addictive part of the tobacco—nicotine—activates certain white blood cells called neutrophils, which in turn release molecules that lead to increased inflammation. This is significant today because while we've known for decades that smoking causes cancer, experts weren't sure why the inflammatory response was so high. Nicotine is the link. Which means that even if you enjoy "safer" alternatives to cigarettes—from smokeless tobacco to cigars you don't "inhale" to cool new stuff like vaping and/or eCigs—if you're ingesting nicotine, you're still triggering an immune response that floods your body with inflammation. Face facts: With tobacco, there's simply no way to win.

---

pain, bloating, and fatigue, and has been connected with all those diseases previously mentioned.

And it gets worse. Not only does food cause inflammation, which can cause weight gain, but the fat you store can itself begin to secrete inflammatory substances —a double-whammy of food-induced inflammation and your body creating it from your belly fat (we'll talk more about this in a second).

You can change this. Researchers are proving time and time again that fitting certain foods into your diet may be all that's needed to counteract the effects of inflammation-perpetuated weight gain. These healing foods attack inflammation by increasing the concentration of beneficial bacteria in your gut, turning off inflammatory switches,

Rethink Hand Sanitizer

You may think hand sanitizer will zap germs and prevent you from getting sick, but if you use it a lot it could also be making you fat. The germ-killing substance contains triclosan, which researchers have found to be an "obesogen," meaning it could cause weight gain by disrupting your body's hormones. A study published in the journal *PLOS One* found that people who had detectable levels of triclosan in their bodies were associated with a 0.9-point increase in their body mass index. Meanwhile, a 2018 study at the University of Massachusetts Amherst found that triclosan raised colon inflammation and altered gut bacteria in mice. Word to the wise for germaphobes looking to lose weight: Rely on good ol' soap and water instead.

---

and decreasing levels of pro-inflammatory biomarkers—many of which will torch fat in the process. Fit these foods into your diet—Chapter 4 is an epic tribute to these foods—and you'll be on your way to a leaner, happier you.

THE INFLAMMATION PROCESS: HOW IT HAPPENS

Chronic inflammation is a complex response, often described as a cascade effect of reactions in the body. Here's a (very) basic breakdown of what's going on:

Something attacks. As previously mentioned, this could be anything from a pathogen (virus, bacteria, parasite) to a physical trauma (cut or bruise, sprain, burns, even frostbite) to a hypersensitivity (allergies). There are many pathways to chronic inflammation. For our purposes, it's lifestyle: food, etc.

The immune system responds. If you recall high school science, the body produces white blood cells (leukocytes) in response to a perceived threat. Certain leukocytes can produce molecules called cytokines, which act as a messenger saying, "Hey, we need some inflammation over here, stat." The body goes into full attack mode with its inflammatory response. Blood is the primary delivery system for all these substances—which is why inflammation can be so pervasive.

The bad guys of chronic inflammation go to work (see page 10). The body continues to respond to "attacks," which in our case is continuous consumption of pro-inflammatory foods, weight gain, sedentary behavior, and rampant stress. Because these lifestyle issues are themselves chronic, the body continues to respond with inflammation. The result is chronic, low-grade inflammation that eventually damages tissues (arterial walls around the heart, for just one example).

I've deliberately simplified the inflammatory process here, as some of the more technical terms for processes and substances are so brutal to the layperson's ear, they'd make any character in a TV thriller say, "Speak English, Doc." (Try these: Cyclooxygenase-1 and Cyclooxygenase-2; we need two because one simply isn't enough.) Some of them are collected and explained in "The Bad Guys of Chronic Inflammation."

The point of all this is simple: When it comes to lifestyle-induced inflammation, you have the power to stop this vicious cycle of tissue destruction. Let's take a closer look at how food in particular wreaks havoc on your weight and digestive system to make inflammation an endless production cycle.

The Bad Guys of Chronic Inflammation

Get to know some of the most common and notorious players in the inflammation game.

Omega-6 fatty acids. Found in most cooking oils, along with salad dressings and mayonnaise, the omega-6 is an "essential" fatty acid (meaning the body needs it to function, but can't make it on its own) and plays a part in the inflammatory immune response. The problem is overconsumption. Too much omega-6 produces inflammation, which is why you'll commonly hear things like, "omega-6 bad, omega-3 good." Not everyone is afraid of it, though. Arachidonic acid is an omega-6 fatty acid used as a supplement by some bodybuilders to promote muscle inflammation, and theoretically, muscle growth.

Trans fats. Trans fats, which are created by partially hydrogenating vegetable oils, are beloved by manufacturers because they increase the shelf life of processed foods, but should be avoided when buying, cooking, or ordering food because of the role they play in weight gain. Trans fats cause inflammation in the body leading to insulin resistance and impairing the body's ability to use glucose properly, resulting in excess fat storage around the belly. (You'll hear more about trans fats in Chapter 3).

Free radicals. Oxidative atoms that are part of the metabolic process and immune response. You can also ingest them via the usual nasty suspects: smoking, unhealthy foods, and alcohol. Too many of these radicals cause oxidative stress, which is a fancy term for cell and DNA damage. Free radicals are linked to premature aging and disease. Antioxidants (see Chapter 2) counteract the effect of free radicals.

Homocystine. An amino acid derived from protein synthesis. Homocystine levels tend to rise in people who eat a heavy protein diet with few fruits and vegetables. Too much homocystine in the blood can cause inflammation and is linked to coronary artery disease. The vitamin B group (including folate) has been shown to lower homocystine levels.

Cortisol. A Good Guy who under normal, healthy circumstances acts as an anti-inflammatory check on your immune system. Lousy circumstances, however, turn cortisol into a Bad Guy. It works like this: When you experience stress or a threat, your body goes into fight or flight mode and releases stress hormones like cortisol, which tries to rein in inflammation and keep your immune system in check. Chronic inflammation, however, keeps cortisol pumping, which naturally messes with your immune system in a big way. Gastrointestinal problems are common under these conditions (in other words, stress and inflammation do a number on your bowels).

Cytokines. Messenger molecules that help regulate the immune and inflammatory response. They can be good guys, or at least just going about their job, but certain cytokines can be responsible for excessive inflammation, such as . . .

Adipokines. Inflammatory cytokines secreted by adipose tissue (a.k.a. fat, particularly visceral, or belly fat) that have been linked to obesity, insulin resistance, type 2 diabetes, and cardiovascular disease. **Interleukin-6 and tumor necrosis factor-alpha** are specific pro-inflammatory adipokines.

C-reactive protein. Produced in the liver and released in the blood as a response when inflammation is detected. That's why it has become a reliable test marker for chronic inflammation.

Advanced glycogen end products (AGEs). Linked to oxidative stress and inflammation, AGEs are produced in heat-processed foods—sugars gone bad, so to speak. Any high-heat cooking technique—from grilling to baking—can produce AGEs in meats and also baked goods. Studies have shown that limiting AGEs in the human diet can help delay chronic disease and aging.

Cyclooxygenase-1 and -2 (COX-1 and COX-2). Enzymes that aid in converting substances like omega-6 arachidonic acid into inflammatory substances. You may have heard of a class of non-steroidal anti-inflammatory (NSAID) drugs called COX-2 inhibitors used to reduce inflammation and pain.

INFLAMMATION, GUT HEALTH, AND BELLY FAT: WHY THE RIGHT FOODS MATTER

Food follows a predictable route: fork, mouth, stomach, and you know the rest. What happens after "stomach" is of particular interest here. By now you surely have heard about "gut health," and how the billions and billions of microbes living in your digestive system—your gut microbiome—have a powerful effect on how your body processes food and even on your overall health. Inflammation plays a big role in your gut health.

It's pretty simple: When you eat unhealthy, inflammatory foods, you starve the good bacteria in your gut. The bad bacteria take over. This balance-imbalance is called dysbiosis. Now, think of the lining of your digestive system like a fine screen (the epithelial lining, to be specific). When bad bacteria start outnumbering the good, the balance falls out of whack, and the bugs begin to irritate the lining of the intestines, and the holes in the screen become larger. Bacteria, food particles, and other nasty things escape your GI tract and get into your bloodstream, where they begin to attack the body. The body fights back with inflammation, leading to weight gain and bloating, and putting you at greater risk for all the health problems we've been talking about.

So that's one nasty way that diet can mess with your health and bring on inflammation. But guess what? If you start putting on weight—due to the inflammatory foods and your body's chronic response, and plain-n-simple overeating—the weight itself becomes an inflammatory issue. Since forever, doctors always thought fat was an inert substance, stored energy. But science has revealed that fat is far from inert. It's metabolically active—and not in a nice way. It releases a type of inflammatory cytokines called adipokines (Bad Guys), particularly interlukein-6 and tumor necrosis factor-alpha. These pro-inflammatory chemicals continue to worsen inflammation, sending you into a waist-widening downward spiral: Bad food, bad bacteria, bad inflammatory reaction, bad weight gain, bad adipokines, more and more inflammation. Then you eat some more bad food, and it all just keeps going.

What's worse, once our belly itself becomes inflamed, our risk rises, most specifically for diabetes. In fact, early in 2015, Australian and Japanese researchers found they could reverse diabetes by dampening the inflammatory response in fat tissues. In a study in the journal *Nature Immunology*, the researchers revealed that in healthy people, fat has its own specialized immune cells, called regulatory T cells, or "Tregs." These Tregs act like guardians of our immune system, protecting us from the inflammation that's related to diabetes and arthritis. But when obesity sets in, the Tregs actually disappear from our fat cells. "The fat tissue of obese people has lower numbers of Tregs than the fat tissue of people in a healthy weight range," the researchers explained. "We can no longer think of fat tissue simply as energy storage. Fat tissue is increasingly being recognized as a crucial organ that releases hormones" and plays a key role in decreasing disease.

If there's any reason at all to attack belly fat and inflammation with food, these last few paragraphs are it. In Chapter 2 we'll take a closer look at why a healthier diet works so well against the inflammatory response (and we'll finally meet some of the Good Guys of Inflammation).

LET'S TALK ABOUT YOUR DOCTOR

A simple statement for clarity: This 14 day program is designed so anyone can try it, but it can be so much more effective and useful if you involve your doctor.

You don't have to, of course. You can skip to the food section, stick to the recommended foods, mix in some recipes, and in two weeks you can tally your weight loss. You can also assess how you feel (probably pretty good). However...

Some things you can't do without your doctor's participation.

Some things you *shouldn't* do without your doctor's participation.

Let's talk about them one by one...

Only your doctor can tell you your inflammation levels and what they mean. Your body's inflammation levels can only be measured by a blood test (see next section for specifics). If you want to know, you have to go. There's no way around it. And once you have those test results in hand? You need a medical pro to interpret them for you. So here's the suggestion:

- Make the 14-day plan part of an overall push to get a handle on your health.

- Set up an annual physical/well visit with your doc.

- When you talk, raise your concerns about chronic inflammation.

- Request that inflammation blood tests be part of the blood panel your doctor would normally prescribe during a physical. (The blood tests are not exotic or expensive.)

Buy a Reusable Water Bottle

Before you begin the habit of refilling your water bottle several times a day, make sure yours isn't laced with BPA (bisphenol A), an industrial chemical used in plastics. A Harvard study found that adults with the highest concentration of this in their urine had significantly larger waists and a 75 percent greater chance of being obese than those in the lowest quartile. Other research has also found a direct link between BPA levels and increased levels of pro-inflammatory cytokines. To avoid inflammation and weight gain, make sure your bottle is BPA-free and be particularly wary of plastics that sport a #7 recycling symbol on them, which is an indicator that BPA may be present.

- Important: Also request that you have a follow-up blood draw in 14 days to re-test your inflammation levels and see how they've changed.

If your doctor is onboard with the plan, you'll have a more complete picture of your overall health—new baselines from the physical, and two-week results after you finish the plan.

Only your doctor can recommend what to do about chronic inflammation. You know your doctor best, but it's possible that when you raise concerns about chronic inflammation, your doctor may make it part of a larger conversation centered around more conventional health data on your chart. For example, the average physician is on the lookout for the big red flags: your weight, blood pressure, blood sugar, cholesterol, family history, and other data that scream trouble if they rise too high. Your doctor may not even consider inflammation as a discussion factor because it's assumed to be part of the bigger package she's already discussing with you. Or if you voice concern about inflammation, your doctor may simply say lose weight, get active, eat better, and the inflammation will improve along with all the Big Red Flag numbers. That's fine. The point is you have to have the conversation. Listen to what your doctor says about inflammation—and the associated health markers—and what to do about it.

Only your doctor can evaluate, diagnose, and prescribe treatment for medical conditions. This is the most important one. The 14-Day Anti-Inflammatory Diet is not a cure for any medical condition. It's designed to help you improve your overall health via healthier eating and making other positive lifestyle changes.

If you're coming to the plan with a pre-existing inflammatory condition, or suspect you may be, for example, an undiagnosed diabetic or pre-diabetic, you need to work directly with your doctor. Many inflammatory diseases, like rheumatoid arthritis, inflammatory bowel disease, and type 2 diabetes may be improved through dietary changes, but any treatment for any condition (diagnosed or undiagnosed) must come from a physician. Example: Many anti-inflammatory foods happen to be fruit, which contain natural sugars. If you're diabetic, your doctor may not want you eating a ton of sugar-laden fruit, no matter how nutritious it may be.

There's more: Medical conditions can be incredibly individual. One person's condition won't be identical to another's. If you suffer from an inflammatory condition, work with your doctor on your unique case and talk about dietary changes that may help. Consulting a registered

Consider Organic

■ Even if you're stocking up on fruits and veggies, buying inorganic may be doing your body a disservice, thanks to the pesticides. They have been linked to inflammatory diseases like lupus and rheumatoid arthritis. They don't do your belly any good, either, as certain pesticides have been shown to poison the mitochondria in your cells so the body can't burn fuel. Unburned fuel, of course, turns to fat.

dietician with a background in inflammatory conditions could help as well.

In the end, there's no substitute for professional help.

HOW TO MEASURE INFLAMMATION

That's the big question isn't it? *How can I tell if I have chronic inflammation?* Unfortunately, the only definitive way to measure inflammation in your body is via blood test. That's why it's so crucial to get your doctor onboard with what you're trying to do. Ideally, you'd have a blood test before you start the plan to establish your baseline, and then another after two weeks to see what kind of progress you've made. None of these tests are exotic or overly expensive. One is even part of the complete blood count (CBC) test panel, so asking your doctor for these tests shouldn't be that big of a deal. But you do have to ask.

C-Reactive Protein (CRP). As mentioned, CRP is an "acute phase reactant" produced by the liver when inflammation rises. Therefore, CRP and inflammation rise in lockstep. This

Could You Have Inflammation?

Can you diagnose inflammation yourself? Short answer: No. Blood tests are the only true way at the moment. However, there are some questions you can answer that may give you an idea that you have chronic inflammation on some level. Answer "yes" to any of these and you should huddle up with your doctor for advice and formal testing.

- Am I overweight?
- Do I carry much of my excess weight around my middle?
- Do I eat a lot of junk and ignore fruits and vegetables?
- Do I spend days at a desk and evenings on a couch?
- Am I tired all the time?
- Am I unhappy, angry, and stressed a lot of the time?
- Do I smoke, drink alcohol to excess, or use drugs?
- Do I have allergies or sensitivities to food or the environment?
- Has my doctor tested me for insulin resistance, metabolic syndrome, or type 2 diabetes?

test can be used to monitor inflammation status over time, as well. Any score greater than 2.0 mg/L is considered high.

Fasting blood glucose and hemoglobin A1C. Insulin resistance is a common marker and/or precursor for type 2 diabetes, which is linked with chronic low-grade inflammation. Also, the adipokines released by belly fat are pro-inflammatory and linked to insulin resistance. While these tests don't indicate precise levels of inflammation, per se, they do indicate that inflammation is present and a serious problem.

Take a Hard Look at "Gluten-Free"

Gluten-free foods aren't all automatically healthy. People with a specific gluten sensitivity have to eat gluten-free by default, but a lot of people who have no gluten issues still go gluten-free for a number of reasons. If that's you, take a closer look at the gluten-free products you buy. People often lose weight and feel better on a gluten-free diet, but it's usually not because of lack of gluten. It's because they're paying attention to their food choices and eating more real foods and fewer simple carbs. If you decide to go gluten-free, read your food labels. Gluten-free packaged foods may have more calories and extra fat or sugar for added flavor.

Other possible blood tests. Red Cell Distribution Width is part of the Complete Blood Count (CBC) panel, and elevated scores can be a marker for inflammation and oxidative stress. Also, serum ferritin, a blood cell protein that stores iron, is an acute reactant like CRP, so elevated levels could indicate inflammation.

Is there an over-the-counter test option? Yes. An OTC urine test is available at ChronicInflammationTest.com for $80. It doesn't measure inflammation directly, but looks at an indirect marker called (this is a mouthful) 11-dehydrothromboxane B_2, which measures thromboxane A_2 production. What does all that mean? Reference your previously mentioned Bad Guys: 11-dehydrothromboxane B_2 is produced by Cox-1 and -2 reactions with the Omega-6 arachidonic acid, which can kick up inflammation. It could be a useful marker along with blood tests, as long as you don't mind sending urine through the mail.

The 14-Day Anti-Inflam

Okay, we've talked all about inflammation and how food and life-style conspire to keep you fat and unhealthy. Let's let the sun come up a bit now. Let's talk about what's to come: An open road leading to healthy weight loss, lower inflammation and disease risk, and feeling terrific. The 14-Day Anti-Inflammatory Diet is a simple program. All you need to do, for two weeks, is accept the challenge and commit to the following steps:

Step 1.
Avoid the foods that have been proven to raise inflammation in the body.

Step 2.
Embrace the foods in chapter 4 that have been proven to combat inflammation and improve gut health (do these first two things alone and you're ahead of most of the population when it comes to improving your life).

Step 3.
- **Eat three meals a day and two snacks.** Chapter 6 can help with planning. Chapters 7 and 8 can help with a big ol' pile of recipes.

natory Diet At a Glance

- **Follow the guidelines on "liquid calories" in chapter 5.**

- **Strive for 7 hours of quality sleep each night.**
  Chapter 10-A has all the details.

- **Engage in some kind of physical activity every day for at least 20 minutes.** Chapter 10-B lists all the options and even has a brand-new fast-and-simple strength workout you can try.

- **Get happy.** Wait . . . is that a trick answer? Nope. You want to focus on this plan. You need to commit to this plan. But there is no reason whatsoever that you can't smile and enjoy yourself on this plan. Have fun. Explore new foods. Take a vacation from your old lifestyle. Consider the *daily* possibility of a new and healthier YOU. If you still feel pressure to succeed, consult chapter 5 for motivational and mindset support. And if you still need some ideas on how to take your stress levels down a notch, yup, we have a chapter for that, too: 10-C.

Now look back at that list. You know what all that adds up to? Taking the next two weeks to regain control of your life, treat your body with respect, and live each day in a reasonable, achievable, simple, and healthy way.

That's worth a two-week effort.

Let's get started.

2

Inflammation, Food, and You

How the food you eat can calm the fire and protect your body for life

NOW YOU KNOW what inflammation is and how it happens. Time to find out what you can do to fight it. The short answer: a lot.

The 14-Day Anti-Inflammatory Diet is all about combating and reversing inflammation in your body with food and weight loss. The good news: Adhering to foods with anti-inflammatory properties makes weight loss simpler because most of them are inherently low-calorie, packed with nutrients, and do everything they can to naturally lower inflammation and reverse your body's tendency to store fat. Just ahead in Chapters 3 and 4, we'll talk in detail about specific foods that cause inflammation and reduce it, respectively. How do they do that? That's what this chapter is all about. Foods can fight inflammation in several ways. We'll look at two of the most powerful: by infusing your body with antioxidants and by improving your gut health.

Adding Antioxidants

You may have heard of antioxidants and free radicals before, and their conflict is one for the ages. This battle is fought on a molecular level. It's pretty simple: Free radicals are created during normal cellular metabolism but are unstable cells that have lost an electron and can damage other cells (free radicals are also known by other names like oxidants and reactive oxygen species). The problem, as with any problem that goes from healthy to unhealthy, is that free radicals are fine until they aren't. For example, your body can marshal free radicals to take on a bacterial attack during the immune response (which is a very interesting link, since chronic inflammation stems from an over-engaged immune system). This can be a good thing. The more common outcome, however, is a body with too many oxidants and too few antioxidants. This triggers *oxidative stress*, which causes nasty damage to your cells, including DNA mutation, and can lead to ugly outcomes like premature aging and cancer.

What causes free radical formation and oxidative stress? No surprises here: External influences include lousy diet, smoking, alcohol abuse, high blood sugar, infections, pollution, and of course, lack of antioxidants in the diet. All classic causes of chronic inflammation.

How are free radicals specifically linked to chronic inflammation? Here's one way: During the immune response, cells like leukocytes (white blood cells) go to work on the threat, which causes the cells to uptake oxygen (they're breathing heavy from the effort). One result is reactive oxygen species production. Inflammatory cells also bring on the cytokines, which continues the process and prolongs inflammation while producing more free radicals. Thus oxidative stress encourages chronic inflammation.

Depending on what kind of movies you like, this is the part where the intrepid group of heroes steps up (war movie, superhero movie, space opera, you pick; cue the horn section): Antioxidants! These Good Guys are able to neutralize free radicals by transferring an electron and stabilizing them. Again, it sounds simple, but understand that all of these processes and reactions and cascade effects happen over and over, and we humans never feel a thing. At least until the damage is bad enough to compromise our health.

There may be one catch, however, before we move on. All of this info might make you think, "If antioxidants are so beneficial, why don't I load up on vitamins and other supplements?" Humans don't get off that easily. Research has shown that high-dose antioxidant supplementation may indeed *cause* oxidative stress. One study in the *Annals of Internal Medicine* reviewed 19 clinical trials with more than 135,000 participants and found that high-dosage vitamin E (a classic antioxidant) raised folks' all-cause mortality risk. Other studies looked at different antioxidants and found similar results. So change your brain from *more must be better* to *too much of a good thing is bad*. Our job is to keep things simple: If you're eating lots of fruits and vegetables, your diet is supplying you with plenty of antioxidant power to counteract all the free radicals, eliminate oxidative stress, reduce chronic inflammation, and protect your cellular health.

We'll take a detailed look at all the terrific anti-inflammatory foods in Chapter 4, but we couldn't wait to tell you about tea. It's that good. Tea—a humble drink that's been cherished as a health miracle for centuries—has been shown time and again to be a powerful anti-inflammatory weapon. Now, for most Americans, tea is tea—that finely ground gunpowder that comes in bags from Lipton, or that over-sweetened sludge sloshed into plastic bottles and sold in between the Coke and the Mountain Dew. However, in places like Japan, the U.K., and large swaths of Southeast Asia, tea leaves are as diverse and nuanced as wine grapes. Not only does the flavor profile change dramatically between one tea variety and the next, but so do the health benefits. One is lower inflammation. Another is weight loss. When Taiwanese researchers studied more than 1,100 people over a 10-year period, they determined that those who drank tea had nearly 20 percent less body fat than those who drank none. Let's take a look at a few common varieties...

Green tea. This cornerstone brew is packed with compounds called catechins, the group of phenols concentrated in the leaves of tea plants that boast robust antioxidant-like properties. And the most powerful of all catechins, a compound called epigallocatechin gallate, or EGCG, is found almost exclusively in green tea. Scientific studies, like one in the *Journal of Advanced Pharmaceutical Technology & Research*, suggest that the high EGCG and polyphenol content in green tea make it a stronger anti-inflammatory elixir than other teas like black tea (although those teas have their benefits, too). Meanwhile, an animal study published in *The FASEB Journal* suggests that EGCG can combat the ill effects of a high-fat and high-fructose diet, which include weight gain, type 2 diabetes, and memory impairment. What's more, the *Journal of Indian Society of Periodontology* report also found that green tea improves lipid and glucose metabolism, prevents blood sugar spikes, and balances metabolic rate. The study also found that green tea's ability to interfere with the body's inflammatory response to periodontal bacteria can help promote oral health while warding off disease.

Catechins can also be belly-fat crusaders that rev the metabolism, increasing the release of fat from fat cells, and then speeding up the liver's fat burning capacity. In a recent study, participants who combined a daily habit of 4 to 5 cups of green tea with a 25-minute sweat session (or 180 minutes a week), lost two more pounds than the non-tea-drinking exercisers. Meanwhile, a research team in Washington found that the same amount of coffee (5+ cups a day) *doubled* their belly fat. There's more: According to a study in the *Journal of Research in Medical Sciences*, 4 cups of green tea a day resulted in a significant decrease in body weight and waist circumference. Not only that, the same *Journal of Research in Medical Sciences* study found that 4 cups of the green stuff daily was shown to reduce systolic blood pressure (about 33 percent of American adults suffer from hypertension).

Matcha tea. Derived from the Japanese tencha leaf and then stone ground into a bright-green fine powder, matcha literally means "powdered tea," and it's incredibly good for you. Research shows the concentration of EGCG in matcha to be 137 times greater than the amount you'll find in most store-bought green tea. You now know that studies have shown the compound can simultaneously boost lipolysis (the breakdown of fat) and block adipogenesis (the formation of fat cells) particularly in the belly. One study found men who drank green tea containing 136 mg EGCG—what you'll find in a single 4 gram serving of matcha—lost twice as much weight as a placebo group (-5.3 vs -2.8 lbs), and four times as much visceral (belly) fat over the course of three months. You can prepare the powder as a traditional tea drink as the zen monks have done since 1191 A.D., or enjoy the superfood modern-style in lattes, iced drinks, milkshakes, and smoothies.

Black tea. Oolong, or "black dragon," is a Chinese tea that's packed with catechins. A study in the *Chinese Journal of Integrative Medicine* found that people who regularly sipped oolong tea lost a pound a week, without doing anything else to change their diet or exercise habits. Meanwhile, Japanese scientists found that high levels of antioxidants called polymerized polyphenols, specific to oolong tea, inhibit the body's ability to absorb fat by up to 20 percent.

There's more: Italian researchers found that drinking a cup of black tea per day improves cardiovascular function—and the more cups you drink, the more you benefit. And a study published in the *Proceedings of the National Academy of Sciences* revealed that drinking 20 ounces of black tea daily causes the body to secrete five times more interferon, a key element of your body's infection-protection arsenal. Just make sure to ditch the dairy. A study in the *European Heart Journal* found that while black tea can improve blood flow, adding milk to the tea counteracts these effects.

Ginger tea. Not only is ginger one of the healthiest spices on the planet, but it also fights inflammation. According to numerous studies, ginger, traditionally used to ease stomach pain, blocks several genes and enzymes in the body that promote bloat-causing inflammation. This means you can enjoy that second serving of nutrient-dense veggies without worry. If you prefer the taste of chai tea, typically made from a blend of cinnamon, cardamom, cloves, and ginger, that may also do the trick—but may be less potent.

Goji tea. We've already extolled the benefits of green and black teas, but research indicates goji tea is another winner. Lycium barbarum, the plant from which goji berries are harvested, boasts a slimming effect. In a study published in the *Journal of the American College of Nutrition*, participants were either given a single dose of L. barbarum or a placebo after a meal. The researchers found that one hour after the dose, the goji group was burning calories at a rate 10 percent higher than the placebo group, and the effects lasted up to four hours. What's more? Most goji teas are mixed with green tea, making the beverage a weight loss double whammy.

Red tea. Rooibos tea, or red tea, is made from the leaves of the "red bush" plant, grown exclusively in the Cederberg region of South Africa, near Cape Town (it's also not technically a tea—it's an herbal infusion). What makes rooibos tea particularly good for your belly is a unique and powerful flavonoid called aspalathin. According to South African researchers, polyphenols and flavonoids found in the plant inhibit adipogenesis—the formation of new fat cells—by as much as 22 percent. The chemicals also help aid fat metabolism. In addition, aspalathin increases stress resistance and promotes longevity under stress according to a study in *Phytomedicine*. Plus, rooibos is naturally sweet, so you won't need to add sugar.

Give it a try: Cook your food in tea. There are so many amazing properties in tea and so many healthy foods that require hot water, so try swapping in hot green tea instead of water for things like oatmeal and quinoa.

We'll dig into more antioxidant-rich foods in Chapter 4. For now, let's talk about the second major way you can use food to fight inflammation...

Improving Gut Health

Another way food can force your body into a state of chronic inflammation is by starving your gut microbiome (bacteria need food, too!). Here's how: Inflammatory foods typically lack natural fiber—a critical nutrient that not only keeps you fuller longer but also feeds your gut bugs. Your good bacteria nosh on and ferment these fibers into a fatty acid—known as butyrate (a Good Guy)—that encourages more efficient fat oxidation. Higher levels of butyrate reduce inflammation in your body and also act as a defense against bad, pathogenic bacteria, according to a review in *Advances in Nutrition*.

There are hundreds of known bacterial species, and a happy gut should have a lot of them. Research is showing that the diversity (both the number of different species and the evenness of those species) of your microbiome is an important part of your health. In fact, a study in the journal *Nature* found that individuals with a low bacterial diversity were characterized by heavier weight, insulin resistance, abnormally elevated cholesterol and lipid levels in the blood, and a more pronounced inflammatory phenotype.

So feeding your gut bacteria with regular doses of fiber—and nutrient-dense foods in general—is critical to reducing overall inflammation. What's more, there is increasing evidence that the composition of our microbial community influences the nutritional value of food. How's that? Isn't food the same no matter who eats it? Not exactly. Our gut bugs help digest and break down the proteins, carbs, and fatty acids in our food so we can extract its nutrients, including essential vitamins such as B vitamins 12 and 9 (folate) and vitamin K. Folate is important for keeping your DNA control mechanisms functioning properly—i.e. keeping your fat genes switched off. In fact, research has shown the *Bifidum* species of bacteria—which is typically lower in obese individuals—is particularly active in producing folate. So, less *Bifidum* means less control over your genes and more belly fat.

Meanwhile, fiber isn't your gut's only friend. You now know that free-radical-fighting antioxidants known as polyphenols are essential in reducing inflammatory oxidative stress, but a study published in the *Journal of Clinical Biochemical Nutrition* found an additional benefit might be due to their contribution to gut health. In rats fed a high-fat diet, only rats who also consumed an anthocyanin polyphenol extract (similar to what you'd find in blueberries) were able to decrease the damaging effect on the rats' gut microbiota. Looking at the results together, the researchers speculated polyphenols may play a significant role in the prevention of degenerative diseases

The Good Guys of Inflammation

Get to know some of the most common and beneficial players in the inflammation game.

Omega-3. The "good" fatty acid. Also, one of the most studied. Omega-3s have consistently been shown to have anti-inflammatory powers and may be protective against our worst health issues. If you don't know already, fish is the most common dietary source of omega-3s. If you choose to take supplements, be sure you pick one labeled "pharmaceutical grade" for quality.

Unsaturated fats. Generally considered the healthy fats (as opposed to saturated and trans fats). Monounsaturated fats (olive oil, avocado, nuts) have been shown to lower the risk of cardiovascular disease, while polyunsaturated fats (fish, flax, oils) include omega-6 and omega-3. As previously mentioned, overconsumption of omega-6 is a no-no.

Fiber. An indigestible carbohydrate. Soluble fiber (oatmeal, beans, blueberries) dissolves in water and can help regulate blood sugar and cholesterol. Insoluble fiber (whole grains, legumes) doesn't dissolve in water and aids in digestion and regularity. As mentioned, fiber also can feed your good gut bacteria to help reduce inflammation.

Antioxidants. Nutrients commonly found in fruits and vegetables that help prevent cell damage via oxidative stress. There are hundreds of types, but well-known examples include vitamin A, vitamin C, vitamin E, lycopene, and selenium.

Polyphenols. A group of phytochemicals found in plants that have been shown to have antioxidant and anti-inflammatory properties. Examples you may have heard of: resveratrol (wine, grapes), catechins (tea, apples, berries), quercetin (onions, broccoli, berries), and curcumin (turmeric).

Butyrate. A beneficial fatty acid produced by fiber fermentation in the gut. Butyrate helps preserve the gut barrier and rein in inflammation.

Rutin. Found in plant pigment, rutin offers antioxidant power and helps your body use vitamin C. Apples, tea, citrus fruits, and bananas are common sources.

(as well as aiding in weight loss) because they improve your microbiome environment.

Now, before we move on, let's talk about a specific kind of fiber that can help turn your gut biome into a bacterial paradise: *Prebiotic.*

Prebiotic / Probiotic: What's the Difference?

They sound alike but are two different things that work together to create a healthy gut biome.

Probiotic: Live bacteria that help promote good gut health. They can be created via fermentation in foods like yogurt, sauerkraut, and kimchi (and can also be taken as dietary supplements). Lactobacillus, which is found in yogurt, is one common example.

Prebiotic: A type of fiber that reaches the lower intestines without being digested, and ferments to help feed beneficial bacteria—including probiotics—in the gut.

Sounds easy, right? Eat plenty of prebiotics *and* probiotics and you're doing a number on bad gut bacteria and chronic inflammation. Just so long as you remember they're a team. It turns out that when you eat probiotics without changing your fast-food, high-carb, and bad-fat diet, it's as useless as drinking decaf coffee during an all-nighter. According to a study in *Science*, probiotics are unable to colonize and mend your gut microbiota when you continue to eat a saturated-fat-heavy, fiber-free, unhealthful diet. So, probiotics don't dig pizza, burgers, and french fries. They're into a fiber-rich, plant-based diet.

When your good gut bugs get the right foods, microbes

can ferment them into short-chain fatty acids like butyrate, compounds which nourish the gut barrier and help prevent inflammation and mend insulin sensitivity—all three things essential for weight loss. They also have the proper fuel to perform other regulatory functions, like keeping your appetite in check and your skin glowing.

Some common foods rich in prebiotic fiber: pulses (beans, peas, etc), dark chocolate, oats, onions, spinach, blueberries, garlic, asparagus, apples, and whole grains (all are among the anti-inflammatory foods in chapter 4). Some of these are hopefully in your kitchen already. But if you want to branch out, try these more exotic prebiotic sources.

Jerusalem artichokes are also known as sunchokes, but they're neither related to artichokes nor are they from Israel. (As it turns out, the green chokes you see in the spring will also provide you with inulin fiber as well—just not as much.) These tubers have a nutty, slightly sweet taste and act as a great substitute for french fries. This type of artichoke is about 76 percent inulin—making them one of the foods highest in this prebiotic fiber.

Dandelion greens. You won't look at these weeds the same way again. That's right. One of the best prebiotic sources for your gut is growing in your backyard. These bittersweet spring greens are bursting with fiber, antioxidants, vitamins, and minerals. And studies have found that this plant is protective against obesity as well as depression, fatigue, and immune system problems because it's a wonderful source of prebiotic fibers. In fact, you'd only need 1 ounce of these greens to provide you with an entire daily serving of fiber. Use them in a salad or steep them in a tea.

Sweating and Sleeping are Good for Gut Microbes

Exercise and sleep can be strong inflammation fighters — lots of details about that in the special section at the end of this book — but since we're on the subject of gut health, the following seemed pretty darn relevant...

Exercise: Not only does exercise help you lose weight by burning off calories, but studies are showing it may also help you torch belly fat by altering the kinds of organisms that live in your gut. A study published in the journal *Gut* examined the differences in the gut composition of athletic rugby players and a group of sedentary, overweight, or obese men. The rugby players had considerably more diversity in their gut microbiomes than the men in the sedentary group, as well as a larger number of Akkermansiaceae, a bacterium that has been linked with a decreased risk for obesity and systemic inflammation. Staying active will also promote healthier digestion, helping your body process, break down, and eliminate food more frequently—which can also aid weight loss.

Sleep: According to a study in the journal *PLOS One*, people who often shift the times they go to bed—essentially living in a state of chronic jet lag—can shift their gut microbiota to an inflammatory state. Respect the ZZZs!

When Anti-inflammatory Foods Cause Inflammation

For anyone who's ever had a bad reaction to eating an otherwise "healthy" food, this section is here to serve as a gentle reminder that when you read about the anti-inflammatory powers of certain foods in this book, we're writing in general terms.

For example: *Generally*, most people can eat apples. Some can't (or shouldn't).

Same goes for any foods containing gluten. Or yogurt for people with dairy issues. Or almonds for people with nut allergies.

The best anti-inflammatory intentions will backfire if you have certain food sensitivities or allergies.

Tennis great Novac Djokevic has famously described the food sensitivities that held him back physically for years. He grew up in war-torn Serbia eating at his parents' pizzeria every day because that's what was available. Later, after going pro, he assessed his diet and went through food sensitivity testing. The results showed how he had specific issues with the three primary pizza ingredients: dough, tomato sauce, and cheese. He'd eaten so much of those things growing up that his body produced an immune response. When he eliminated those foods from his diet, he felt physically transformed. His new nutrition approach elevated his physical abilities, and he eventually became the number one ranked player in the world.

The point is, you may not be a pro athlete, but food sensitivities are highly individual and can cause an inflammatory response in your body. If you suspect you have an undiagnosed food sensitivity, get tested. Or, more simply, avoid that food and see how you feel. Our bodies are goofy machines sometimes. The only way to figure them out is to keep trying new and different things so that even when things get goofy, we can still make it all work in our favor.

Shake the Salt

Your body needs sodium, sure, but most of us eat way too much, and too much salt causes inflammation in your body. A 2018 study in *Joint Bone Spine* found that salt may provoke an autoimmune response, raising inflammation, in people with inflammatory conditions like lupus, multiple sclerosis, and colitis. Another study that fed adolescents more than double the recommended intake of salt—3,280 mg/day—resulted in higher inflammation levels, and the salt-inflammation link has also been found in adults. One British study found that for every additional 1,000 milligrams of sodium you eat a day, your risk of obesity spikes by 25 percent.

So, avoid salting your food and be wary of the sodium content in restaurant fare and manufactured food products. Food manufacturers and restaurants engage in salt overkill. When we eat processed foods and restaurant fare, we're taking in far more than the recommended 2,000 mg/day for adults. Here's one example: The Crispy Chicken Club Sandwich with Croutons and Ranch Dressing at Jack in the Box delivers 1,980 mg, nearly your total sodium for a day, in just one meal. And we've become accustomed to sodium overload even in places we least expect to find it (a 1 cup serving of Cheerios, for example— a seemingly innocent breakfast cereal— has comparable amounts of sodium to a small bag of Lay's potato chips, 160 mg to 170 mg). If you want to cut back on salt, cut back on eating out. And when you make food at home, check those nutrition labels.

3

Foods that Fan the Flames

The science behind junk food and inflammation (and why you need to avoid these foods like the plague they are)

IF THERE ARE two sides to every story, here's side one: Certain foods cause inflammation. Side two—foods that cool inflammation—comes in the next chapter. The math is pretty simple: See fire, add gas, watch fire go *whooooosh*. In other words, if you want to reduce inflammation in your body, don't let it get inflamed in the first place.

As you read this collection of inflammation-causing foods, you'll no doubt notice a running theme in all of them: They are the general ingredients in heavily processed, unhealthy fare—sugary, fatty, calorie-laden stuff that's frighteningly free of nutrients.

But that's what makes them so hard to shake! These

are the foods that are engineered to be irresistible to the human palate—perfect, lab-rendered balances of salt, sugar, and fat to produce brain-teasing flavors that can quite literally become addictive. And the terrifying cycle begins: Empty calories in, your body responds, inflammation stirs, fat is stored, that fat produces even more inflammation, and your brain says "That was good; bring me more!"

Use this list as a weapon, for as you read, you'll begin to see how these substances do their best to totally toxify your body. Think about that the next time you see your favorite tempting processed food.

Added Sugar

Bet you could've guessed this one. According to a review in the *Journal of Endocrinology*, when we eat too much sugar, the excess glucose our body can't process quickly enough can increase levels of proinflammatory messengers called

32

Teaspoons of added sugar the average American consumes each day, according to the USDA

cytokines. And that's not all. Sugar also suppresses the effectiveness of our white blood cells' germ-killing ability, weakening our immune system and making us more susceptible to infectious diseases. A simple swap is subbing out harmful high-glycemic (GI) foods (which spike and crash blood sugar) for low GI alternatives, like whole grains and foods with healthy fats, protein, and fibers. A study in the *Journal of Nutrition* discovered that on an equal calorie diet, overweight participants who ate a low-GI diet reduced levels of the inflammatory biomarker C-reactive protein while participants on a high GI diet did not. Sugar isn't only added to obvious products like candy bars and sodas. It's also lurking in foods marketed as "healthy," like yogurt. (See our list in "The Added-Sugar Hall of Shame," page 42.)

The American Heart Association recommends no more than 100 calories per day from added sugars, or six teaspoons, for women, and 150 calories (nine teaspoons) for men. And those recommendations make complete sense: New research suggests that for every 5 percent of total calories you consume from added sweeteners, your risk of diabetes increases by 18 percent. That's scary because it doesn't take much added sugar to do damage. The average woman consuming 1,858 calories a day only needs to eat 93 calories of added sugar to significantly boost her risk.

Alcohol (overdoing it)

We're suggesting you abstain from booze for the 14-Day Anti-Inflammatory Diet, but alcohol is worth discussing so you understand how it affects you if/when you do drink. While some research has shown a drink a day can actually lower levels of the inflammatory biomarker C-reactive protein (CRP), too much alcohol has the opposite effect. That's because the process of breaking down alcohol generates toxic by-products that can damage liver cells, promote inflammation, and weaken the body's immune system. On the other hand, the flavonoids and antioxidants found in wine—as well as the probiotics in beer—might contribute an anti-inflammatory effect, according to a study published in the journal *Toxicology*. We can't say it enough, "Everything in moderation!" *Common Culprits: beer, wine, and liquors.*

The Added-Sugar Hall of Shame

The Expected:
- Soda
- Candy
- Baked sweets
- Desserts
- Coffee drinks
- Breakfast cereals
- Toaster pastries
- Table syrup
- Fruit juices
- Hazelnut spreads

The Unexpected:
- Yogurt
- Oatmeal
- Canned vegetables
- Canned beans
- Tomato sauce
- Smoothies
- Sports drinks
- Energy drinks
- Protein powders & bars
- Hot dogs & sausages
- Salad dressing
- Seasoned nuts
- Peanut butter
- Bread
- Dried fruits
- Pasta
- Ketchup, BBQ, and other sauces
- Wine
- Frozen meals

Artificial Additives

This is a big one because these substances are found in so many processed foods. Artificial means not found in nature. And that means your body usually doesn't have a way to process it. Ingredients like artificial coloring—which are made from petroleum (oil)—have been implicated in a host of health issues, from disrupting hormone function, to causing hyperactivity in children, to tumor production in animal studies. And a meta-analysis in the journal *Alternative Therapies in Health and Medicine* found that our immune system attempts to defend the body from these synthetic colorants, which activates the inflammatory cascade. Another study by researchers at Georgia State University found that additives like emulsifying agents used to thicken foods can disrupt the bacterial makeup of the gut, leading to inflammation and weight gain in animals. The evidence in humans is sparse, but your best bet would still be to steer clear of these ingredients, and stick to their natural counterparts. *Common Culprits: breakfast cereals, processed foods containing fruit, candy, ice cream.*

Artificial Sweeteners

A 2014 study published in *Nature* found that artificial sweetener consumption in both mice and humans enhances the risk of glucose intolerance by altering our gut microbiome. Researchers also found an increase in bad gut bacteria that had previously been associated with type 2 diabetes. When our bodies can't metabolize glucose properly, it can lead to a greater release of inflammatory cytokines, as is the case with sugar and refined carbs. On top of that, artificial sweeteners disrupt the composition of our gut microbiota by decreasing levels of the good

Choose Your Beef Wisely

If beef is your preferred source of protein, make sure you're eating the grass-fed stuff. Ground beef, a T-bone steak, or prime rib are among the healthiest cuts because they're lower in unhealthy fats than other forms of beef, and grass-fed varieties may contain more heart-healthy omega-3 fatty acids than some fish. Just be sure to limit your red meat consumption to around two 3-ounce servings per week, and stick to low-calorie rubs and spices as opposed to sugary sauces to flavor the meal.

---

bacteria *bacteroides*, which are known to help release anti-inflammatory compounds. Consider: In a 2012 study in *The American Journal of Clinical Nutrition*, researchers found that those who drank diet beverages had higher fasting glucose, thicker waists, lower HDL (good) cholesterol, higher triglycerides, and higher blood pressure. *Common Culprits: no-sugar-added products, no-calorie "diet" soft drinks.*

Conventional Grain-Fed Meats

Because cattle, chicken, and pigs didn't evolve on a grain-fed diet, many producers have to load up their animals with antibiotics to keep them healthy. These drugs not only keep the animals from getting diseases in cramped feedlots or getting sick from their unnatural diet, but they also help them (and us) gain weight faster. Altogether, this means we're eating meats that are higher in inflammatory saturated fats, have greater levels of inflammatory omega-6s from the corn and soy diet, and our body thinks it's in a constant state of attack due to ingesting leftover levels of antibiotics and hormones. Even worse, when we grill meat at high temperatures, it creates inflammatory carcinogens. Besides limiting red meat to fewer than three days a week, make sure you pick up lean cuts of grass-fed beef for your protein. This healthy source provides healthier saturated and trans fats as well as inflammation-fighting omega-3s. And you can also add a bit of lemon juice to your meats—the acid acts as an antioxidant, protecting you from the harmful carcinogens produced during grilling. *Common Culprits: beef, chicken, pork.*

Dairy

While moderate consumption of yogurt can actually help decrease inflammation with its gut-healing probiotics, dairy is also a source of inflammation-inducing saturated fats. On top of that, studies have connected full-fat dairy with disrupting our gut microbiome, and decreasing levels of our good gut bacteria, which are key players in reducing inflammation. And lastly, dairy is a common allergen, with about 1 in 4 adults having a difficulty in digesting milk, whether it's lactose intolerance or a sensitivity to its casein proteins. Either way, any type of allergen can trigger inflammatory reactions through the release of histamines. If you feel particularly bloated after a few blocks of cheese, you might consider cutting dairy from your diet. P.S. Don't worry about not getting enough calcium if you cut out dairy: A 2014 study published in the *British Medical Journal* found no correlation between fewer bone fractures and dairy consumption. *Common Culprits: milk, soft cheeses, butter.*

Fast Food

Even if you don't know how to pronounce it, you should know what phthalates (thāl-ates) are. That's because many of us are unknowingly eating this class of endocrine-disrupting chemical toxins. Similar to BPA, phthalates are used in plastic food and beverage packaging—and they're not staying there. Recently, a study made headlines for finding that people who often ate fast food had dose-dependent higher levels of phthalate metabolites than infrequent eaters of fast food. Bad news for all-day-breakfast lovers since a separate study published in *Environmental Science & Technology* found phthalates to be associated with the CRP marker of inflammation, and another study in *Environmental Health* connected higher exposure to phthalates with metabolic syndrome, a disease also commonly associated with increased levels of inflammation. If all that isn't enough, well, cue Mom: Fast food isn't good for you. *Common Culprits: you know...*

Fried Foods

Another issue with these vegetable-oil-fried and processed foods is that they contain high levels of inflammatory Advanced Glycation End products (AGEs), compounds that form when products are cooked at high temperatures, pasteurized, dried, smoked, fried, or grilled. Researchers from the Mount Sinai School of Medicine found that when people cut out processed and fried foods that have high levels of AGEs, markers of inflammation in their body diminished. *Common Culprits: fried foods like french fries, fried chicken, fish sticks, chicken tenders, onion rings.*

Gluten from Store-Bought Bread

Many of the breads on the market can go from flour and yeast to baked bread in just a few hours. But this shortening of the period of fermentation causes a decrease in the amount of starch and gluten the yeast typically can pre-digest for us. Without the assistance in digestion, it can be harder for our bodies to digest the bread's gluten, causing inflammation in the lining of your intestines. Experts believe this could be one reason for the rise in gluten sensitivity among Americans. Another theory is that modern strains of wheat contain a super starch known as amylopectin A, which has been shown to have inflammatory effects. Either way, store-bought breads should be a pass if you've been struggling to lose weight. We are, however, giving bakery-made sourdough the green light; sourdough bread is one of the surprising fermented foods that provides healthy probiotics to help heal your gut—a key in helping to reduce inflammation. *Common Culprits: store-bought bread made from refined, white flour.*

Refined Flour

Refined wheat flours have been stripped of their slow-digesting fiber and nutrients, which means your body can break down the foods made from this ingredient very quickly. The more quickly your body digests glucose-containing foods, like these carbs, the faster your blood sugar levels can spike, which also increases your insulin level—a hormone associated with a pro-inflammatory response. A *Journal of Nutrition* study found that a diet high in refined grains showed a greater concentration of the inflammatory marker, PAI-1, in the blood. On the other hand, a diet rich in whole grains resulted in a lower concentration of the same marker as well as one of the most well-known inflammatory biomarkers, C-reactive protein (CRP). *Common Culprits: pizza, white bread, crackers, pasta, pretzels, flour tortillas, breakfast cereals, bagels.*

Saturated Fats

We may have just absolved saturated fats of their connection to heart disease, but that doesn't mean they're out of the woods just yet. That's because multiple studies have connected saturated fats with triggering white adipose tissue (fat tissue) inflammation. This white tissue is the type of fat that stores energy, rather than burns energy like brown fat cells do. And as your fat cells get bigger with greater intakes of saturated fats, they actually release proinflammatory agents that promote systemic inflammation, according to a review in the journal *Expert Review of Cardiovascular Therapy. Common Culprits: burgers, pizza, candy, chips.*

Processed Meats

Processed meats are the worst of both worlds. They're typically made from red meats high in saturated fats, and they contain high levels of advanced glycation end products (AGEs), inflammatory compounds that are created when these processed meats are dried, smoked, pasteurized, and cooked at high temperatures. Not to mention the fact that these sometimes "mystery meats" are injected with a slurry of preservatives, colorings, and artificial flavorings that also register as foreign attackers to our immune system. *Common Culprits: bacon, hot dogs, bologna, sausage, jerky.*

All Inflammation-Boosting Foods Have Something Terrible in Common

It's very simple—and scary when you think about it. All of these foods contain virtually zero nutritional value. Think about that. These are some of the most enthusiastically consumed foods (or ingredients in foods) in our culture *and they have virtually no nutritional value.* They bring nothing good for our bodies to use. That's why you hear phrases like "junk food" and "empty calories." Those descriptions are accurate.

We consume these foods in huge quantities for one reason: Taste. That's it. They taste good on their own, or sugar, fats, and salt have been engineered together with other chemical ingredients to be addictively delicious. So there's an argument to be made: What makes them any different than cigarettes? Or an addictive drug? If you wouldn't consider smoking or doing hard drugs, why would you eat something that is designed to have the same effect on your brain while wreaking havoc on your health?

Something to think about.

Trans-Fat Foods

Because manmade partially hydrogenated oils, also known as trans fats, do not occur naturally in foods, our body doesn't possess an adequate mechanism to break them down. And when our body senses an unknown, foreign object, it can stimulate an inflammatory response. According to the Mayo Clinic, trans fats can cause inflammation by damaging the cells in the lining of blood vessels. And a study in the *American Journal of Clinical Nutrition* found that women who ate foods high in trans fat also had higher levels of markers of systemic inflammation, like interleukin 6 (IL-6) and C-reactive protein (CRP). Because the FDA's guidelines allow products with less than 0.5 grams of trans fats to claim 0 trans fats, be sure to read labels and look out for products with partially hydrogenated oils—like almost all of Dairy Queen's blizzards. *Common Culprits: margarine/ shortening; baked goods like doughnuts, cookies, and muffins; non-dairy coffee creamers; frozen pizza; frosting.*

Vegetable Oil

Once we became aware of the artery-clogging ill effects of trans fats, manufacturers switched to injecting their products with or frying their foods in vegetable oils such as soy, corn, sunflower, safflower, or palm oil—which wasn't much better. That's because these vegetable oils have a high concentration of the inflammatory fat omega-6 and are low in the anti-inflammatory fat omega-3. In fact, Americans are eating so many vegetable-oil-laden products that the average person has an omega-6 to omega-3 ratio of around 20:1 when it should be 1:1. To ward off inflammation, ditch the unhealthy oils. We'll show you some healthy oil alternatives in the next chapter. *Common Culprits: mayonnaise, salad dressings, barbecue sauce, crackers, bread, potato chips.*

Foods that Douse the Flames

They're low-calorie, nutrient-dense, and packed with fiber. All you have to do is eat them

"DIET" HAS TWO MEANINGS. It could be a plan you follow, like what's in this book. But it's also something bigger: The entirety of what you eat. That's your diet, and for this chapter, that's how we're going to define the term. The idea here is simple. The more foods you add to your diet—the entirety of what you eat—that are proven inflammation fighters, the better off you'll be. Your body will lower or reverse its inflammation levels, which will help you to lose weight.

This collection of inflammation fighters is meant to serve as a series of ideas—and you'll see these ideas come together to form even more ideas in Chapter 8. The more eating ideas and options a person has in front of them, the better choices he or she will make. Think about it: If you pack your fridge and pantry with tasty healthy choices, you'll crowd out the tasty unhealthy choices. Success sometimes depends on the unhealthy stuff being too much of a pain in the butt to get in the car and seek out! You'll find lots of other ideas throughout this book—the recipe section, for sure, and the sample eating plan in Chapter 6, as well. And the chapter before this one was all about the *lousy* ideas. All these are designed to help you answer the eternal question, "What should I eat?"

Is this collection of foods complete? Probably not. Science is ever-changing, and we learn more and more about food and our bodies through research over decades. But these foods and their ingredients have been studied and found to help people battle chronic inflammation.

There are some very good foods in here, but are there any surprises? Perhaps not. The only thing that's brain surgery is brain surgery, and it's no stretch to say anti-inflammatory foods are classically healthier fare. The key is understanding why and how these foods calm the inflammatory response. By understanding that, the next time you're presented with a food choice—one healthy, one not so much—you'll have so much more data informing your choice. Again, the more healthy options you have, the easier it is to make that good choice. So read on, and choose wisely...

Apples

In order for your probiotic efforts to succeed, you also have to incorporate foods known as prebiotics into your diet. This group of high fiber foods provides your gut bugs with

Forget Fruit Juice

While you might not think there's a huge difference between eating a whole piece of fruit and drinking fruit juice, nutritionally speaking, the two entities are most definitely not one and the same. Whereas whole fruit contains naturally occurring sugars and fiber that can help counteract the bad effects of too much sweet stuff, fruit juice is often loaded with added sugar (such as high-fructose corn syrup) and no fiber to speak of. According to a study led by Harvard School of Public Health researchers, eating more whole fruits, particularly blueberries, grapes, and apples, was significantly associated with a lower risk of type 2 diabetes. On the other hand, a greater consumption of fruit juices was associated with a higher risk of type 2 diabetes.

the fuel they use to function and ferment. Apple peels are full of pectin, a natural fruit fiber that a study published in the journal *Anaerobe* found to be powerful enough to support the growth of the beneficial bacteria *bifidobacteria* and *lactobacillus*. Not to mention, apple peels also provide an average of 10 mg of quercetin, an endurance-boosting, anti-inflammatory antioxidant.

Asparagus

This early-spring favorite doesn't just herald beautiful weather, it's also rich in the flavonoid rutin. A 2014 study in *Inflammation Research* found that rutin may help suppress the production of known inflammation boosters like tumor necrosis factor-a and interleukin 6.

Avocado

Though avocados get a bad rap for being high in calories, they're actually loaded with heart-healthy monounsaturated fats that make you feel less hungry. Need proof? A study in *Nutrition Journal* found that participants who ate half a fresh avocado with lunch reported a 40 percent decreased desire to eat for hours afterward. What's more? Unsaturated fats, such as those found in avocados, have been linked to preventing the storage of belly fat. Avocadoes may also help counteract the inflammatory effects of other foods. A 2013 study in the journal *Food & Function* looked at the amount of inflammation that followed eating a hamburger with and without the addition of avocado. Researchers found that eating the hamburger with about 2 ounces of avocado limited the inflammatory response seen after eating the hamburger alone.

Avocado Oil

Avocado oil is super versatile and delicious. Unlike a lot of oils that are pressed from a seed, avocado oil is made of the same creamy goodness that makes guacamole. This heart-healthy oil has anti-inflammatory properties that help prevent arterial damage, heart disease, and blood pressure. A 2014 study in *Disease Markers* found that avocado oil had a positive effect on C-reactive protein (CRP), a common inflammation marker. It's great in the kitchen, too: You can easily cook with it and make just about anything because of its high smoke point.

Bananas

Monkeys know what's good for them. Bananas are rich in rutin, an anti-inflammatory flavonoid. On top of that, a study in the journal *Anaerobe* found that women who ate a banana twice daily before meals for two months reduced belly bloat by 50 percent. Researchers believe this is because bananas are packed with potassium, which can reduce water retention. The yellow fruits are also a good source of fiber, which will keep you feeling full.

Beets

Besides being a source of many phytochemicals, including ascorbic acid, carotenoids, and flavonoids, beets are a unique source of betalain pigments, which have been found to display potent antioxidant, anti-inflammatory, and chemopreventive activity. One of these pigments, betaine, is a nutrient that not only fights inflammation, but also is known to rev your metabolism, positively influence the mechanism for insulin resistance, boost your mood, and shut down genes that encourage fat to hang around. A review in the journal *Nutrients* has associated eating beets with lower levels of inflammatory markers—including CRP as well as interleukin-6 and tumor necrosis factor, which are released by harmful belly fat—as well as a decrease in risk of plaque buildup, high blood pressure, and type 2 diabetes. Other root vegetables—carrots, turnips, and the like—are fine inflammation fighters, too. They're naturally gluten-free and are loaded with antioxidants and fiber.

Black Beans

Similar to raw oats, black beans and most other pulses pack a strong resistant-starch punch (so let's give other **beans**, **lentils**, **split peas**, and **chickpeas** some anti-inflammatory respect), providing the source of fuel for your healthy gut bugs to ferment into the inflammation-reducing fatty acid butyrate. A half-cup of black beans not only packs 3.1 grams of resistant starch, it also carries nearly 20 grams of protein and 14 grams of filling fiber, making black beans a delicious fat-fighting triple threat. Not only that but black beans are high in anthocyanins, antioxidants which have also been associated with lowering inflammation. According to a recent study in the journal *Nutrients*, when patients with metabolic syndrome consumed a meal with black beans, their levels of postprandial insulin (i.e. those measured right after a meal) were lower and antioxidant concentration higher than subjects who ate a meal with a similar amount of fiber or a similar amount of antioxidants. High levels of postprandial glucose and insulin have been implicated in increases in inflammation and oxidative stress—making black beans a potent Western-diet inflammation-fighter.

Blueberries

A study in the *Journal of Nutrition* showed that eating berries daily could significantly reduce inflammation. And another study in the same journal found that fruit-based drinks could neutralize the inflammatory effects of high-fat, high-carb meals. Why is this exactly? Well, berries contain a class of antioxidants called flavonoids, but it's the anthocyanins, specifically, that contribute their anti-inflammatory effects by effectively turning off the inflammatory and immune genes. And when it comes to anthocyanins, blueberries are king. On top of that, blueberries are rich in vitamin C and another polyphenol, resveratrol, which have both been found to promote anti-inflammatory responses through decreasing free radicals.

Bone Broth

Don't dismiss bone broth as just another health fad—there's solid evidence to back up its rightful place in your diet. To make it, bones are left to simmer in water for an extended

More About Berries

Berries are more than just morsels of sweetness that you can toss on yogurt or work into a smoothie; they can help you lose weight, too! Raspberries pack more fiber and liquid than most other fruits, which boosts satiety. They're a rich source of ketones, antioxidants that can make you slimmer by incinerating stored fat cells. And like other berries, raspberries are loaded with polyphenols, powerful natural chemicals that have been shown to decrease the formation of fat cells and eliminate abdominal fat. Not to be outdone, research suggests blueberries can also help blast away stubborn belly fat by engaging your get-lean genes. After a 90-day trial, University of Michigan researchers discovered rats that were fed a blueberry-enriched diet showed significantly reduced belly fat compared to those who skipped the berries. Whether you pick rasp-, blue-, straw-, or any other kind of berry, you can't go wrong.

---

period of time, extracting and breaking down their collagen and other nutrients. Some of that broken down material from the cartilage and tendons is glucosamine (which you may have seen sold as a supplement for arthritis and joint pain). According to a study published in the journal *PLOS One*, when overweight, middle-aged adults took a glucosamine supplement, they were able to decrease serum CRP (inflammation biomarker) levels by 23 percent more than those who didn't take a supplement. The stock is also full of anti-inflammatory amino acids (glycine and proline), and the ample levels of gelatin will help rebuild your gut lining to further assist with your anti-inflammatory gut microbes.

Broccoli

This anti-inflammatory benefit could be linked to the

sprouts' glucosinolate content. These compounds help prevent unwanted inflammation when they're converted to I3C—a compound that research has found to decrease the production of pro-inflammatory mediators on a genetic level. It's also high in vitamin K, a vitamin found in many cruciferous and leafy green veggies, which can help regulate inflammatory responses in the body.

Brussels Sprouts

In addition to serving up nearly two days' worth of cortisol-fighting vitamin C, this cruciferous veggie is a good source of heart-healthy omega-3s. If you don't care for fish, sprouts and other foods rich in the nutrient like walnuts and flaxseeds are important additions to your diet.

Canned Light White Tuna

According to a 2016 study published in the *American Journal of Clinical Nutrition*, the most effective omega-3 when it comes to reducing specific markers of inflammation is DHA over EPA. So, how do you get more of the powerful fat into your diet? It's easy (and cheap)—just grab a can of light skipjack tuna, which is one of the best sources of the bioactive fatty acid.

Canola Oil

With any oil, the key to consider is its ratio of omega-3 (anti-inflammatory) to omega-6 (inflammatory) fats. Canola has a near-even ratio of the two, which has shown to help battle cancer, arthritis, and asthma. It's also gleaming with Alpha-Linolenic Acid (ALA), an essential omega-3 fatty acid that may play a role in weight maintenance.

This is the good option for everyday cooking, as it can

What About Tuna Salad?

Who doesn't like a tuna sandwich? The trouble is all that mayonnaise. It's a calorie bomb and tastes so good you always want more (yes, you do). For the 14-day plan, let's keep the tuna and ditch the mayo. Here are two healthy and incredibly delicious alternatives:

Salsa. Mix a can of tuna with salsa and you add anti-inflammatory vegetables without the calorie load. And they pair as well as PB&J.

Balsamic vinegar. Flaked tuna on a bed of arugula drizzled with balsamic is a fantastic lunch. And again, you avoid all those mayo calories.

---

endure relatively high levels of heat and has a neutral flavor that won't overpower a dish. Penn State researchers found that canola oil may also stimulate weight loss. After one month of adhering to diets that included canola oil, participants had a quarter-pound less belly fat than they did before the diet. They also found that the weight lost from the midsection did not redistribute elsewhere in the body. Like avocados, canola oil's belly-blasting abilities are thought to be a result of the monounsaturated fats it contains.

Cauliflower

There's so much you can do with cauliflower. You can make a low-carb rice out of it, mash it, or even turn it into crispy buffalo wings. And the more you use it, the more you'll benefit from its anti-inflammatory mix of antioxidants.

Chia Seeds

With 9 grams of healthy fats (including inflammation-quelling ALA omega-3s) alongside a whopping 11 grams of fiber and 4 grams of protein per ounce, chia seeds can stabilize blood sugar, boost weight loss, suppress appetite, and even help keep your body hydrated throughout the day. Put them all together, and you have an inflammation-fighting superfood. According to a study in the *European Journal of Clinical Nutrition*, loaves of bread supplemented with increasing doses of chia seeds were found to decrease spikes in blood sugar in a dose-dependent manner. Post-eating blood sugar spikes have been implicated in increases in inflammation due to the overproduction of inflammatory free radicals called reactive oxygen species (ROS).

Cinnamon

Cinnamon is loaded with antioxidants, so it's a well-known inflammation fighter. Also, research from the University of Michigan Life Sciences Institute has determined that the popular holiday spice can help fight obesity thanks to cinnamaldehyde, an essential oil that gives cinnamon its flavor. According to researchers, cinnamaldehyde improves metabolic health by acting directly on fat cells, inducing them to start burning energy via thermogenesis. To work cinnamon into your diet, try sprinkling some on oatmeal or sipping on cinnamon tea.

Cilantro

Cilantro, though polarizing in terms of taste, contains a unique blend of oils that work much like over-the-counter meds to relax digestive muscles and alleviate an "overactive" gut. A study published in the journal *Digestive Diseases and Science* found that patients with IBS benefited from supplementing with cilantro as opposed to a placebo because their bellies weren't as bloated.

Citrus Fruits

Oranges, grapefruit, tangerines, lemons, and limes are all powerhouse sources of vitamin C and antioxidants. They're also simple to incorporate into your day. Not only is drinking lemon water, for example, a healthy, low-calorie alternative to soda or juice, but lemons themselves have also been shown to contribute to weight loss. Just one of the citrus fruits contains an entire day's worth of vitamin C, a nutrient that has the power to reduce levels of cortisol, an inflammatory stress hormone that triggers hunger and fat storage. Additionally, lemons also contain polyphenols, which researchers say may ward off fat accumulation and weight gain. Believe it or not, even the peel is beneficial because it is a potent source of pectin—a soluble fiber that's been proven to help people feel fuller for longer. According to a study published in the *Journal of the American College of Nutrition*, participants who ate just 5 grams of pectin experienced more satiety. A longtime vitamin C MVP, the orange is a good source of fiber and potassium, and rich in cancer-fighting citrus limonoids, too. Add oranges to a smoothie, stir pieces into Greek yogurt, or eat the whole fruit on the run for a perfectly self-contained, de-stressing snack. As for grapefruit, try it as an appetizer. A study in the journal *Metabolism* found that eating half a grapefruit before meals may help reduce belly fat and lower cholesterol levels.

Coffee

Your morning java contains polyphenols that may have anti-inflammatory properties. That's good. What's bad? All the stuff we put in coffee to make it taste better: dairy creamers, artificial flavors, and lots and lots of added sugar.

If you take your coffee black, good for you. All that other stuff? Bad for you.

Dark Chocolate

Great news for all you chocoholics! A recent study found that antioxidants in cocoa prevented laboratory mice from gaining excess weight and lowered their blood sugar levels. And another study at Louisiana State University found that gut microbes in our stomachs ferment chocolate into heart-healthy, anti-inflammatory compounds that shut down genes linked to insulin resistance and inflammation. And how about this: A study among women with normal weight obesity (or skinny fat syndrome) who ate a Mediterranean diet that included two servings of dark chocolate each day showed a significant reduction in waist size than when on a cocoa-free meal plan. To enhance the effects, try pairing your chocolate with some apple slices: The fruit speeds up the probiotic fermentation process, leading to an even greater reduction in inflammation and weight. *Psst*, make sure you're choosing the right kind! Look for cacao content of 70 percent or above because these contain the highest amounts of antioxidants.

Eggs

Besides keeping brittle bones at bay, vitamin D also fends off depression and colds, reduces the risk of certain cancers, and perhaps most importantly, diminishes inflammation. Previous research has found a correlation between vitamin D deficiency and increased levels of pro-inflammatory markers. While your body produces D whenever your skin is directly exposed to sunlight, if you've been finding that you're glued to your desk more often than you'd like, it might be best to get some vitamin D into your diet as well, and whole eggs are a great solution. The yolk contains a host of fat-blasting nutrients from vitamin D to choline.

Worried about cholesterol in eggs? Don't be. The Dietary Guidelines Advisory Committee dropped their longstanding recommendation that we should limit dietary cholesterol. Decades of research have shown that it has little effect on blood cholesterol levels, and the government's outdated recommendations have done little more than send scrambled messages about the pros and cons of eating eggs. So go ahead and scramble up an omelet—with the yolk.

Extra Virgin Olive Oil

Add fighting inflammation to the list of Mediterranean Diet benefits—right next to reducing the risk of cardiovascular disease and dialing up weight loss. While researchers initially believed many benefits were conferred by the presence of healthy monounsaturated fats, they also found that other oils with MUFAs, particularly oleic acid, did not exhibit the same health benefits. Now, researchers have found the key component is oleocanthal. This compound, found only in extra virgin olive oils (as these are unrefined and contain more phenolic compounds), has a significant impact on inflammation and helps reduce joint cartilage damage, working similarly to ibuprofen in that it prevents the production of pro-inflammatory COX-1 and COX-2 enzymes.

Flaxseed

Flax is a potent source of omega-3s, which makes it especially valuable if you don't like fish. But the real inflammation-fighter in flax may be lignans. Chances are you haven't heard of lignans, but the plant compounds found in flax seeds (and sesame) have been shown to help reduce the action of some genes that cause inflammation. In a 2015 study, women who consumed high levels of lignans tended to weigh less and gain less weight over time when compared to women who didn't consume these compounds in high amounts. Flaxseeds can pass through your body undigested, so grind them up and add them to smoothies, cereal, yogurt, or salads.

Garlic

There's now science to back up the smelly, cold-busting benefits of garlic. Researchers hypothesize garlic's cold-fighting power comes from the compound allicin, which blocks enzymes that play a role in bacterial and viral infections. In terms of an inflammatory response, a review in *Anti-Cancer Agents in Medicinal Chemistry* explained that aged garlic extract has been found to favorably stimulate anti-inflammatory proteins while suppressing markers in chronic inflammation environments. Taking an aged-garlic supplement provides the highest concentration of bioavailable compounds, but studies have also shown that fresh garlic can provide benefits. Just be sure to crush the garlic first to kickstart production of the bioactive allicin compound. There's more: A 2016 study found that garlic powder reduces body weight and fat mass among people with non-alcoholic fatty liver disease (NAFLD). Recent studies have also shown that garlic supports blood-sugar metabolism.

Ginger

Researchers attribute ginger's surprising health benefits

Swap Veggies for Cheese in Your Omelet

If you're accustomed to shredding muenster cheese into your eggs, try swapping it out for your favorite veggie. One ounce of cheese packs in about 110 calories while a half cup of steamed broccoli boasts 15 calories. Making this morning switch will nourish your body with extra satiating fiber and nutrients, as well as save your waistline from added inches.

to gingerols, key compounds that are antioxidant, anti-inflammatory, antibacterial, and anti-disease. According to numerous studies, these compounds block several genes and enzymes in the body that promote inflammation. When University of Arizona researchers gave rats with experimental rheumatoid arthritis a crude ginger extract, which included the essential oils and other compounds found only in the root itself, it was able to inhibit joint swelling and inflammation. Fresh ginger is richest in gingerol, so grate up the root, throw it in a mesh bag, steep, and sip on ginger tea.

Herbs

Popular herbs like basil, rosemary, and sage have strong anti-inflammatory properties, which is terrific news as they have so many uses in the kitchen. Too many food options is never a bad thing!

Kamut

There's a new superfood in town, and its name is kamut—or Khorasan wheat. This ancient grain boasts more protein gram-for-gram than quinoa, it's loaded with energy-boosting, muscle-protecting minerals like magnesium, potassium, and iron, and comes complete with an amazing 7 grams of hunger-busting fiber per cup. Plus, a half-cup serving of the stuff has 30 percent more protein than regular wheat and only 140 calories. A study published in the *European Journal of Clinical Nutrition* found that noshing on Kamut reduces cholesterol, blood sugar, and cytokines (which cause inflammation throughout the body). Subbing out meat for plant-based vegan foods is great for reducing inflammation because animal protein is one of the top sources of inflammatory saturated fats.

Kiwi

They may be small, but these sweet-tasting fruits with the brown skin contain a hefty amount of actinidin, a natural enzyme unique to kiwifruit that aids in digestion by breaking down protein in the body. Kiwifruit also contains prebiotic fiber, which primes the gut for healthy digestion. Research indicates that a daily serving of green kiwifruit helps increase bowel movements. So, cut one in half, scoop with a spoon, and pop into your mouth like nature's Tums (SunGold kiwis, with a yellow flesh and tropical taste, offer three times the vitamin C of oranges and as much potassium as a medium banana).

Miso

Miso packs an anti-inflammatory one-two punch. Not only is it a fermented food, which means it's rich in probiotic compounds that ferment fibers into anti-inflammatory compounds, but it's also made from soy. What's so special about soy? Several studies have suggested that soy's isoflavones—estrogen-mimicking compounds—may be powerful anti-inflammatories. A review of isoflavones published in a 2016 issue of the journal *Nutrients* concluded that isoflavones reduce inflammation by reducing pro-inflammatory enzyme and cytokine activities.

Nuts

Although not as strong as animal-based omega-3s, DHA and EPA, nuts (particularly walnuts) are a great source of a plant-based, anti-inflammatory omega-3 known as ALA. Almonds are one of the best sources of antioxidant vitamin E, which helps protect cells from oxidative damage (a byproduct of inflammation), and hazelnuts contain the highest amount of immuno-protective oleic acid. Meanwhile, walnuts may help reduce the inflammation that comes with allergies. According to a 2017 study published in the *Journal of Clinical Investigation*, the high amount of omega-3s in the nuts can help reduce symptoms.

Oysters

Healthy nutrients like copper can help maintain anti-inflammatory and antioxidant responses in the body. That's because this essential mineral acts as a critical cofactor in the body's anti-inflammatory responses. The enzyme superoxide dismutase (SOD) plays an important antioxidant role in deactivating cell-damaging free-radicals. And in order to function properly, it utilizes the support of three minerals: copper, zinc, and manganese. And guess what? Oysters are full of all three. Oh, not to mention, they're also a great source of inflammation-quelling omega-3s.

Pineapple

Pineapple contains bromelain, the enzyme which acts as a meat tenderizer as well as a powerful anti-inflammatory. What researchers have noted is that many anti-inflammatory foods act not necessarily by reducing inflammation directly, but by alleviating symptoms that can eventually cause inflammation. Bromelain has been found to be beneficial in reducing asthmatic symptoms through decreasing the spread of pro-inflammatory metabolites and relieving post-exercise inflammation by helping to repair and resolve muscle soreness through its significant levels of potassium. While all parts of the pineapple contain this magical compound, most of the bromelain in pineapple is in the stem. Because the stem is a little on the tough side, you can blend or juice the core with the sweeter flesh to reap the bloat-beating benefits.

Pomegranate

Not only is pomegranate packed with fiber (which is found in its edible seeds) but it also contains anthocyanins, tannins, and high levels of antioxidants, which research published in the *International Journal of Obesity* says can help fight weight gain. A half-cup of the colorful fruit gives you 12 grams of fiber and more than half a day's vitamin C. Snack on these fruits raw or toss 'em into a smoothie, and you're good to go.

Quinoa

As far as grains go, quinoa is a great one to have around if you're looking to lose weight. It's packed with protein and fiber, and contains approximately 220 calories per cup, cooked. What's more? Quinoa is one of the few plant foods that offer a complete set of amino acids, meaning it can be converted directly into muscle by the body. It's also incredibly versatile and can be eaten as part of a salad, tossed in a smoothie, or on its own as a side dish.

Raw Honey

If you've ever suffered from indigestion after eating, you're familiar with the importance of digestive enzymes. But there's another group of enzymes that's also important to your health: proteolytic enzymes. These enzymes are essential when it comes to modulating the inflammatory response. They do so by helping to break down proteins and cellular debris and clear them out to reduce your body's immune and inflammatory response. Raw honey is one of the best sources of these enzymes because—brace yourself—honey is made by bees' enzyme-rich saliva. Multiple animal studies have found honey to be effective in alleviating symptoms of inflammatory diseases, such as IBS. Bonus: The sweetener is also full of anti-inflammatory polyphenols, carotenoids, antioxidants, and vitamins.

Raw Oats

Throw together a jar of overnight oats packed with dark chocolate, berries, nuts, and a dash of cinnamon, and you'll be fighting inflammation and drastically reducing belly fat. The raw oats are a resistant starch, a type of carb that passes through your gut undigested. Instead of feeding you, it feeds your healthy gut bacteria, which in turn produce a fatty acid that encourages more efficient fat oxidation known as butyrate. Higher levels of butyrate reduce inflammation in your body and help reduce insulin resistance as well. Less inflammation means less bloating and a slimmer you.

Red Cabbage

Add a cup of shredded cabbage into a salad and you'll add 66 percent of your daily allowance of vitamin C, as well. And if you decide to boil it, you'll unlock a waterfall of inflammatory-fighting antioxidants as well.

Red Grapes

Red grapes are easy to love: they're delicious, make for a quick portable snack, and *always* hit the spot. They're also rich in the anti-inflammation helpers flavonoids and resveratrol. One study also found that their polyphenols may help prevent you from coming down with seasonal allergy symptoms.

Red onions

Onions, particularly the red variety, are loaded with flavonoids, particularly quercetin, an anti-inflammatory that has been shown to reduce histamine response, as well as inhibit inflammatory leukotrienes. They're a handy ingredient because they go so well with so many meals.

Red Peppers

Peppers are an anti-inflammatory superfood—but go red to reap the most benefits. Out of the three colors of bell pepper, red have the highest amount of inflammatory-biomarker-reducing vitamin C, along with the bioflavonoids beta-carotene, quercetin, and luteolin, according to research in the *Journal of Food Science*. Luteolin has been found to neutralize free radicals and reduce inflammation. Beta-carotene is a carotenoid, a fat-soluble compound that is associated with a reduction in a wide range of cancers, as well as reduced risk and severity of inflammatory conditions such as asthma and rheumatoid arthritis. And allergy research has shown that quercetin acts as a mast-cell stabilizer, which decreases the number of cells reacting to an allergen. Mast cells are responsible for releasing histamine during inflammatory and allergic reactions.

Rosemary

It's not just a staple when you're marinating your lemon chicken; this flavorful herb is also a powerful anti-inflammatory thanks to its high concentration of antioxidant compounds. (In fact, you'll often see "rosemary extract" listed on your natural processed goods as an antioxidant preservative.) Scientists believe the anti-inflammatory activity comes from the presence of carnosic acid and carnosol, two polyphenolic compounds in rosemary which a study published in the journal *BMC Complementary and Alternative Medicine* discovered could effectively inhibit the production of pro-inflammatory cytokines.

Saffron

As far as spices go, saffron is one of the most expensive ones around, but it's also a substance that preliminary research suggests can contribute to weight loss. According to a study published in the journal *Antioxidants,* saffron extract may inhibit weight gain in a number of ways similar to how antioxidants function. The research suggests the colorful spice could decrease calorie intake by blocking dietary fat digestion, act as an antioxidant and suppress inflammation, suppress food intake by increasing satiety, and enhance glucose and lipid metabolism. Though scientists aren't totally sure what makes saffron so weight-loss friendly, they suspect it has something to do with crocetin and crocin—two antioxidant-rich compounds found in saffron that give it its distinct color.

Soy

Soy looks to be a strong anti-inflammatory food, which is a good thing because edamame and tofu are so versatile in any diet. A study of 1,005 Chinese women in the *Journal of the Academy of Nutrition and Dietetics* found that soy consumption lowered levels of inflammatory markers like interleukin-6 and tumor necrosis factor-alpha. Soy is high in polyunsaturated fats, fiber, and isoflavones and has also been shown to reduce production of inflammatory cytokines.

Spinach

Spinach attacks inflammation from all sides. It's rich in carotenoids and vitamins C, E, and K—all of which have been found to protect the body from pro-inflammatory cytokines. A form of vitamin E called alpha-tocopherol was found to decrease inflammation in patients with coronary artery disease in a *The American Journal of Clinical Nutrition* study. And in a separate study in the *Canadian Journal of Surgery*, vitamin E administration was found to reverse levels of the same inflammatory adipokine compounds released by belly fat: tumour necrosis factor-a and interleukin-6.

Sweet Potato

Think of sweet potatoes as nature's dessert. Not only do they satisfy your sweet tooth, these taters digest slowly and keep you feeling fuller for longer thanks to their satiating

Hot Peppers: How to Fight Fire with Fire

It may sound counterintuitive, but while spicy peppers raise the temperature in your mouth, they douse inflammation in your body. A compound called capsaicin gives peppers their heat—the hotter the pepper, the more capsaicin it contains. For years, studies have found positive analgesic and anti-inflammatory benefits in capsaicin. What's more, hot peppers are a terrific dietary delivery method. They don't just bring the heat; colorful peppers also mean antioxidants. Plus, some research has found that people who consume a spicy meal may end up consuming fewer calories overall, as capsaicin may also aid satiety. Spice up your menus and enjoy the benefits!

fiber. They're also brimming with carotenoids, antioxidants that combat inflammation, stabilize blood-sugar levels, and lower insulin resistance—which prevent calories from being converted into fat.

Tart Cherries

Tart cherries are grown exclusively in Michigan, but if you're able to get your hands on them there is strong evidence to suggest they can help you achieve your weight loss goals. Need proof? Researchers at the University of Michigan conducted a 12-week study that found that rats fed tart cherries showed a 9 percent belly fat reduction over those fed a standard western diet. Scientists believe this is because tart cherries are especially high in anthocyanins, a type of flavonoid with strong antioxidant activity. These and other flavonoids found in tart cherries have also been shown to have anti-inflammatory effects.

Tomatoes

Since tomatoes can be grown indoors, they never really go out of season, making them a reliable weight-loss staple to add to your diet. Tomatoes are a great source of lycopene, an antioxidant that protects your brain and fights depression-causing inflammation. Because lycopene lives in tomato skins, you'll get more of the stuff if you throw a handful of cherry tomatoes into your next salad instead of slicing up one full-size tomato. And if you're not a fan of the tart, raw tomatoes, don't sweat it; research has proven that processed tomatoes have an even higher amount of lycopene than the fresh ones. Whatever your choice, enjoy them with a little olive oil, which has been shown to increase fat-soluble lycopene absorption. More food for tomato thought: They have a high water content, and they're low in calories. A study published in *Nutrition Journal* found that eight weeks of tomato juice consumption helps the body burn about an additional 100 calories per day.

Turmeric

You can thank curcumin for turmeric's beautifully bright, yellowy-orange color—but that's not all it's good for. This active compound has been found to contain potent anti-inflammatory and antioxidant properties. Studies

SEE RED: Red fruits such as watermelon, Pink Lady apples, and plums have higher levels of nutrients called flavonoids— particularly anthocyanins—compounds that give red fruits their color, which have been shown to reduce fat-storage genes.

Add Some Apple Cider Vinegar

According to a study published in *Bioscience, Biotechnology, & Biochemistry*, consuming apple cider vinegar each day can lead to weight loss, reduced belly fat, waist circumference, and lower blood triglycerides. More specifically, the study of obese Japanese participants found that those who consumed just one tablespoon of ACV over a three-month period lost 2.6 pounds, and those who consumed 2 tablespoons lost 3.7 pounds in the same time frame. ACV is considered an anti-inflammatory by many (it is derived from apples, after all). Go ahead and toss a tablespoon or two of this calorie-, fat-, and sugar-free stuff in your next salad dressing, sauce, or smoothie.

have shown curcumin directly inhibits the activation of inflammatory pathways through shutting off production of two pro-inflammatory enzymes, COX-2, and 5-LOX. For this reason, curcumin has been touted for a range of beneficial health effects, from preventing cognitive decline, liver damage, and heart disease, to easing joint inflammation and pain associated with arthritis. In a 2015 study in the journal *Clinical Nutrition*, researchers gave 117 patients with metabolic syndrome either supplements of curcumin—the active ingredient in turmeric—or a placebo. Over eight weeks, those who received the curcumin saw dramatic reductions in inflammation and fasting blood sugar.

Whole Grains

Brown rice, millet, and amaranth are all packed with fiber that helps produce butyrate, a fatty acid that turns off genes related to inflammation and insulin resistance. The high B vitamin content of whole grains (which is nearly entirely

Fish for More Seafood Options

We've been clear on the benefits of wild salmon, but those pink creatures are quite literally not the only fish in the sea. Generally speaking, fish provide one of the best sources of fatty acids known as omega-3s, which will help fend off waist-widening inflammation and are an excellent source of high-quality, lean protein. This allows them to help you maintain muscle mass, thus reducing excess fat accumulation. Some of our favorite healthy seafood include mussels, Atlantic mackerel, halibut, and bluefish.

lost during the refinement process) also helps reduce the inflammatory hormone homocysteine in the body. Not only that, high fiber foods suppress appetite. According to a team of researchers, a molecule called acetate is released when fiber is digested. Acetate then travels to the brain, where it signals us to stop eating. And if you eat less, you're less likely to be taking in more pro-inflammatory foods.

Wild Salmon

When it comes to fats, there's one variety you definitely don't want eat less of: omega-3s! These healthy fats are famous for their anti-inflammatory properties. And fatty fish are one of the best sources of this class of polyunsaturated fats. Wild salmon provides you with both EPA and DHA. And unlike plant omega-3s, these two fatty acids are already in an active form, meaning they'll more efficiently attack excess inflammation through the increase in adiponectin—a hormone that enhances your muscles' ability to use carbs for energy, boosts metabolism, and burns fat—which ultimately decrease inflammation markers.

Marinate Meat In Beer

Alcohol isn't a weight loss ally, but using it to flavor meat when you cook it could help you drop a few pounds and stay healthy. Polycyclic aromatic hydrocarbons (PAHs) are nasty substances that can form when meats are cooked at very high temperatures, like on a backyard grill. According to a study in the *Journal of Agricultural and Food Chemistry*, if you marinate meat with beer for four hours, you can lower the harmful chemicals it produces when exposed to high heat by up to 68 percent.

Also know that not all salmon is created equal. Farmed salmon, which is what's commonly sold in restaurants, can have the opposite effect on your waistline. Farmed salmon has over 100 more calories and nearly twice as much fat as wild-caught salmon. Plus, it's much higher in saturated fat and lower in heart-healthy omega-3s. When dining out, skip the salmon unless you're sure it's wild-caught.

Yogurt

Cultivating a proper gut garden is essential for good health, particularly when it comes to fighting inflammation. That's because your good gut bugs break down foods into anti-inflammatory fatty acids, which not only decrease inflammation but may also help shut off your fat genes. And when they aren't healthy, they can't do this. Adding cultured, fermented foods—known as probiotics—into your diet can recolonize your gut with beneficial microbes, which can then assist with fending off inflammation. Low sugar yogurt (with live active cultures) is one of the most accessible sources of probiotics, but you can also eat kefir, sauerkraut, pickles, kimchi, and cheese.

5

7 Smart Success Secrets

**The right mindset will make
the 14-Day Anti-Inflammatory Diet
even easier**

THIS IS AN important chapter. Every other chapter offers crucial information about how to reduce inflammation and lose weight, but none of those chapters talk about what's going on in your brain. Your brain is Grand Central Station for things like motivation, accountability, willpower, and weakness. All of those things track into your *mindset*.

Developing the right mindset is critical for making any positive lifestyle change. You've probably heard it stated different ways: Find your "why," for example. Maybe you want to lose weight for an upcoming event, or you want to feel better, or someone close to you had a very serious health scare (or maybe you did, too). Maybe the thought of a future being overweight, with inflammation pushing your body toward its inevitable health apocalypse, is enough to make you say "enough."

Your "why" is your trigger. After all, I'd bet that you know all about the "secrets" to weight loss and good health. They're not secrets at all: Eat healthier foods in sensible amounts; move more; respect sleep; address stress; and even more basic things like love your family and friends. But here's the catch: You—and millions of other people just like you—know all these things up and down, left and right. You hear them continuously. And yet you have a brutal time trying to lose weight or stick to an exercise plan. Why? Here's where my 20 years of experience working as a health journalist comes into play. Every person I've ever encountered who has successfully lost the weight they wanted and kept it off, or set a fitness goal and hit it and set new goals and hit them, has had one thing in common. At some point, something pulled an emotional trigger within them and they finally used all that knowledge they'd picked up over the years to make things happen. They got to work. They found their "why." Or their "why" was shoved in their faces, and they got the message via heart attack or the sudden death of someone close to them.

You have the knowledge. But knowledge without that emotional trigger is almost always useless. Once something pulls your trigger, you're ready.

Now, you're here reading this book, and you've come this far. So I'll make a bet that your emotional trigger has been pulled to some extent. That's good. This chapter isn't about your "why." You've found your why, and if you haven't, you probably know what it is deep down and haven't admitted it to yourself.

The why is the beginning. The why gets you moving. But *mindset* will keep you moving. That's what this chapter is all about.

Mindset is your approach. It's your day-to-day. It's where you are mentally and how you feel. It's what you tell yourself in moments of weakness—and strength. Mindset keeps you focused. It helps you prioritize. It's not your trigger, or your why, but you can use your why to help reset your mind.

So, in this chapter I'm going to take you through seven very different areas of mindset. Some are straight-on motivation, others about a goal. Some are clear advice about specific situations you'll face as you use the 14-Day Anti-Inflammatory Diet plan. But each one is designed to help you stay on track and improve your mindset as you go. Maybe this chapter can be the positive voice in your head, or the place you return to for a booster shot of confidence. However you use it, keep using it. Because like I said, a good mindset is the one thing I've seen that separates the successful from the unsuccessful. So let's get going...

MINDSET, STEP 1

Commit only to 14 days.

This is the simplest step, but crucial. Set your mind to 14 days. That's it. Two weeks. But *how* you think about these two weeks will determine not just whether you stick to the plan, but if you enjoy it. If in any little corner of your brain you think of these two weeks as some kind of prison sentence, you're in trouble. However, if you think of the next two weeks as a vacation from your old lifestyle, from the things that never worked, or classify it as a new adventure, you're going in with the equivalent of a cool breeze at your back. That's mindset. You set your mind. *You*. Two weeks is a choice and a commitment and it can be wonderful or terrible. *That's* your real choice here.

Some things that might help you along the way:

Announce it. Let your loved ones know that for the next two weeks, things will be different. You'll be embracing new foods and new ways of thinking about lifestyle. Ask for their support. Heck, ask them to join you. But be sure everyone knows that the next two weeks are non-negotiable. You're committing to a plan and that's that.

Document it. Social media can be a pit of slime, as we all know, but it can also help you keep your mission at the forefront of your mind and attract supportive people along the way. Whatever your favorite platform—Facebook, Twitter, Instagram, Reddit, and more—you can find groups of healthy people doing exactly what you're doing. Meal photos are the biggest social media cliché of them all, but if you use those photos as reinforcement, to project your enthusiasm, your progress, you might find that incredibly helpful for your mindset.

Let your mindset be contagious. If people know you're on a new 14-day plan and see you smiling and having a blast, that matters. Good vibes are just as contagious as bad vibes. The difference is that good vibes attract people. The happier you are, the more support you'll receive. Something to think about.

Why stop here? When the 14 days are up, you'll have a lot to review. How much weight did you lose? If you're working with your doctor, what do your new inflammation stats look like? Most important of all, how do you feel? Then set your mind for the next round. A week? Another two weeks? Six months? Your choice. You can go one day at a time, too. But after these first 14 days you'll have had a real taste of not just what a healthy lifestyle feels like, but a healthy mindset. My guess is you'll feel stronger. Happier. Energized. And my guess is you'll want to keep going.

MINDSET, STEP 2

Define what "healthy" really means to you.

This plan is all about losing weight and lowering inflammation. And you can certainly do that. Chances are you want to do that because you want to be healthier. But when you say those words in your mind, "health" and "healthier," what are you thinking about? That's what I mean when I say define what healthy means to you. Is it thin? Or muscular? Easy on the eyes? Or maybe it's more about the numbers—having healthy blood pressure and blood sugar numbers. For people who have already had health problems, maybe it means simply being free of pain and discomfort, or medication, or physical limitations.

That's why "healthy" is such a loaded word. It can mean a lot of different things to different people. But "healthy" or "healthier" can be a legitimate goal for you, and this plan is a start. So from a mindset standpoint, it could be helpful for you to give this some thought. Consider these questions:

If your goal is "healthy," what does healthy look like *to you*?

What does strength look like? How will sticking to this plan for two weeks make you feel strong? How can you use that as motivation?

What does weakness look like? What will you do if you feel weakness when it comes to lousy food or unhealthy habits? How will you prepare for that?

If you're able to answer these questions in your own unique way, you'll go into this plan with the same preparedness as, say, a film director who has storyboarded every shot before production even begins. You have a *vision* of what you want and what you'll want to happen when things get harder. You'll be able to say with certainty, *this* is healthy, *this* is what I want.

Because let's be honest. Saying, "I'm stronger, I'm healthier, I can do this" is a lot better for your mindset than saying, "I'm a snowball in Hell. Pass the Oreos."

Beware the Saboteurs

Sabotage comes in many forms: Someone tempts you with unhealthy food, or peer pressures you about going out for drinks and apps, or wants you to do something other than your scheduled workout, or feels like you're neglecting them because of your new habits and schedule. And there's more: Your closest loved ones could sabotage you because they don't like the food you're preparing, or feel like you're moving in a different direction, or don't understand how much this 14-day challenge means to you. How do you handle these situations? Or other situations where people try—consciously or unconsciously— to knock you off-track?

Well, think about it this way: These people, no matter if they're doing it deliberately with malice or accidentally with no evil intentions whatsoever, are making it about themselves. That's just how most people roll. Everyone is the hero of their own story. You need to be the hero of yours. All you have to do is, gently and simply, make the situation about you. Remind people...

- **You're doing this plan for two weeks.**

- **You're committed to it.**

- **It's nothing personal (Aunt Edna hates when people turn down her chocolate bundt).**

- **You'd appreciate their support.**

That last bit, delivered in the wrong tone of voice, may put off someone who would prefer the situation remain focused on them. Be sweet, patient, and firm. Set your mind. Remember why you committed to the plan in the first place. If necessary, repeat the above statements. In the end, saboteurs are just noise. It really is all about you. But then your final choices are all on you, too.

MINDSET, STEP 3

Know before you go.

This is a more practical, situational tip, but it's important and goes right to successful mindset. This book is loaded with food and recipe ideas, which covers you at home, but what happens in the next two weeks if you're invited to a party or restaurant or picnic or any occasion where you'll have zero control over what foods are served?

Know before you go. It's a simple matter of preparation. Five minutes, tops.

Ask simple questions when you're invited. If it's a party or dinner, "What are you serving?" If the menu doesn't jibe with your plan, you can very nicely say, "You know, I'm really committed to this 14-day thing. Is it okay if I bring a dish?" Who could say no?

As for restaurants, *Eat This, Not That!*—the bestselling book series—as well as EatThis.com—have mastered the fine art of the healthy restaurant swaps based on what was, at one point, information hidden from the public: calorie and nutrition numbers of chain restaurant meals. Now most chain restaurants make their numbers available, even if you have to hunt for then. And you can, but that's not necessarily the problem. Restaurant fare—even something that sounds relatively tame like grilled chicken—is generally prepared with many ingredients you'll avoid during your 14 days: butter, sugar, salt, and unhealthy oils you can't identify from your table in the corner. We say *know before you go,* and you simply can't know what's in the food at most restaurants. So what to do? Change your mindset and don't be afraid to ask your server a few quick, key questions: *How is this prepared? Can you hold the sauce?*

For the Next Two Weeks, Homemade's Better

A 2014 study in the journal *Public Health Nutrition* asked people to report their food intake over the course of two days. Those who ate at a restaurant during that time took in an average of 200 calories per day more than those who prepared all their own meals, and those who ate in sit-down restaurants consumed slightly more calories than those who ordered from fast-food joints.

When dining out, people also consumed more saturated fat, sugar, and sodium, so eating at home where you can prepare food in a healthier way is obviously the better choice.

And ordering take-out to eat at home isn't any better just because you're eating the food at your kitchen table. Research suggests that just the mere presence of take-out food increases your risk of being over-weight. One study printed in the *British Medical Journal* found that just having a lot of take-out options near your work or along your commute to work makes you twice as likely to be obese. Though you obviously have little control over what kind of establishments populate where you live and work, this is just another reason to avoid eating their food. When you prepare your meals at home, you have much more control over the satu-rated fat, sugars, sodium, and calories you consume.

Put the dressing on the side? These may seem like obvious, common sense questions but how many times have you ever asked them while dining out? The whole point is about transferring as much control over what's in your meal from the kitchen staff to you. Consult the online menu at home; make choices and ordering plans ahead of time; know before you go.

Of course, another option for your two-week commitment would be to not go to any restaurants and bring your own dishes to other events. That's legit—it's only two weeks. But it will do your mindset some good to, again, think about all possibilities before you start.

MINDSET, STEP 4

Operate on the fringe.

Of the supermarket, that is. This is another one you may have heard a hundred times, but again, this goes to mindset. As consumers, we're very used to doing the same thing over and over, and changing a big habit to help change an overall lifestyle—even for just two weeks—is a challenge.

Here's the thing, and there's no way around it: If you want to use food to lower inflammation, the foods you need are generally fresh (with certain exceptions like canned tuna, for example, or a bottle of olive oil). Fresh fruits, fresh vegetables, fresh fish and poultry. You'll find them on the periphery of your supermarket. The middle aisles feature a lot of the foods you don't want: packaged, processed foods high in added sugar, salt, and chemicals. The stuff that helped inflame you in the first place.

Oh, and it's worth mentioning something else. The packaged stuff in the middle aisles tends to be a lot cheaper than the fresh, healthier foods. That's a big issue for people. So how do you break the attraction to the center aisles of the supermarket? Well, step back and open your mind to change your mind.

First, commit to the periphery of the supermarket for two weeks. Yes, it may be more expensive, but it's just two weeks for now. But let's think about this less as some cumbersome burden to bear for two weeks and call it what we called it before: an adventure. A two-week break from the same-old thing (that wasn't working well for you anyway).

Wrap your brain around it this way: In the middle aisles, would you ever see something you don't know or haven't tried? Pretty much the best you can say is that manufacturers occasionally add some variation to the shelf: tri-colored pasta, a new flavor of instant oatmeal, and one I'm still waiting for, double-stuff Pop-Tarts. But really, what's on those shelves to be excited about?

The fringe, however, is a wonderland: fruits and vegetables you've never sampled, varieties of fish you've never dared try, different cooking combinations of fresh ingredients. How about the farmer's market? You can talk to the vendors about something you've never seen before. How to cook it? What does it go well with?

For two weeks, you can be an explorer. Or not! You can prep basic salads every day, put a lean protein on top, and have an apple for dessert and still be rewarded with weight loss and lower inflammation.

The point is, how you mentally approach the supermarket matters. Take a two-week vacation from brightly colored boxes of stuff. Try brightly colored fresh things. Try *new* things. After all, habits are all in your head.

MINDSET, STEP 5

Think before you drink.

The 14-Day Anti-Inflammatory Diet deals in liquid calories, but only certain kinds. Chapter 7, for example, is all about smoothies, which are a terrific way to add convenient, powerful anti-inflammatory foods to your day without a lot of effort.

The problem lies with all the other "liquid calorie" possibilities that permeate our lifestyle. You need to set your mind to shun for some of them. Let's start with the big one: alcohol.

You can make an argument for including alcohol in the 14-day plan. Plenty of research has shown that a drink a day for women and two for men may have protective properties when it comes to heart disease and other health issues. Wine in particular—containing resveratrol, a proven anti-inflammatory—can be an asset. You get no argument from me about the positive power of moderate alcohol consumption. However...

I advise leaving booze out of the picture for two weeks for two reasons.

First: the liquid calorie angle. If you have one or two drinks a day—moderate, responsible consumption—you're still adding 100 to 300 calories a day to your total (possibly more, depending on what you drink). Over two weeks, that's 1,400 to 4,000+ calories total. Experts generally accept that 3,500 calories equals one pound of fat, so you're talking about an amount of calories that could affect your bottom line. Ask yourself: Are a couple of drinks a day worth it?

Second: stopping at one or two drinks. For some people, it's like stopping at one or two potato chips. Ain't gonna happen. Here's what does happen. Consume more than two drinks and you're edging into inflammation territory. Yes, alcohol consumed in excess raises inflammation levels (really, does that surprise you?). Also, have a few drinks and what do you want to do (aside from skinny-dip)? *Eat.* Eat snacks and apps and stuff that you swore you would avoid for two weeks. You can add hundreds of garbage calories to your daily total *in minutes.* A *Journal of the Academy of*

Nutrition and Dietetics study found that alcohol causes people to eat an additional 384 calories per day on average, likely because beer, wine, and cocktails make us more sensitive to food aromas and less likely to resist indulgent fare.

So...it's two weeks. Let's just leave booze out of it. As Forrest Gump said, *One less thang.*

Here are some other sources of liquid calories you should avoid for the next two weeks:

Soda. I'd hope this is an obvious one, but some people really love their Mountain Dew (let's include *energy drinks* in this category while we're here). Look, the calories are one thing, but they come strictly from added sugar, which is gasoline to inflammation. If that isn't enough, I'd like to illustrate just how brutal regular soda is to your body. Consider this: When a doctor suspects her patient could be diabetic or on the road toward the condition, she can order an Oral Glucose Tolerance Test, which measures how well your body processes sugar. It works like this: You guzzle a sweet glucose drink containing about 75 grams of sugar. The doctor takes blood glucose readings before and after to see how your body responds. Basically, it's a stress test for some of your most stressed organs. Here's the catch: A 20-ounce regular soda, depending on the brand, has anywhere from 65 to 77 grams of sugar. So if you drink a 20-ounce bottle, you're basically subjecting your system to an Oral Glucose Tolerance Test *every single time.*

Diet soda. Wait, what? Diet soda has no added sugar and no calories. Everybody knows that. True enough. However, diet soda contains artificial sweeteners. And we know from

Chapter 3 that artificial sweeteners can be inflammatory. If you drink diet soda on this plan with the no-sugar/no-calorie argument, you still lose.

Dairy milk. Yes, cow's milk is loaded with nutrients. But remember Chapter 3: regular dairy can act as an inflammatory. Even if something is generally nutritious, why drink it if it will work against your ultimate goal?

Fruit juices. A glass of orange juice is packed with vitamins— particularly vitamin C—which is a known inflammation fighter. What's the problem? With fruit juices you're also getting a bunch of calories without other whole fruit benefits like fiber. If you're going to take a natural sugar hit, make sure it's as close to nature and nutritionally dense as possible. Whole fruit is just better than juice. Also, other fruit juices like apple and cranberry usually come with a dose of added sugar. Lots of wondering, lots of label reading. For two weeks, leave the juices in the fridge.

So...what can you drink?

For two weeks, set your mind to simplicity when it comes to beverages.

Water and sparkling water are simplest (a slice of citrus fruit for flavor is nice). Unsweetened iced tea is a refreshing, no-cal way to get anti-inflammatory antioxidants. *Nut milks* are fair game, too, but be very careful about sweetened/ unsweetened. Added sugar is off limits. You can also sample *vegetable juices* like V8, though I will suggest you stick to the low-sodium versions. And as previously mentioned, hot coffee and tea – without the sweet and creamy add-ins that turn them into sundaes.

Forget Those Unhealthy Food Videos

■ Thanks to an increased interest in food and food trends, recipe videos are likely dominating your social media feeds. And their constant presence could be hindering your weight loss goals, especially since many of the brief clips spotlight unhealthy dishes and sweets. Tomorrow is always another National (Insert Food Here) Day. If you know these clips will get you thinking tempting thoughts, avoid your usual online food haunts for two weeks.

MINDSET, STEP 6

Think beyond food.

Making a two-week commitment to changing your relationship with food is a big thing, but it doesn't have to be the only thing. This chapter is about mindset, and if you want to reset how you think about health and your lifestyle, expand your boundaries to take a more holistic view.

Food can fight inflammation. That much we know. But food ties into our entire lifestyle, and it turns out that other critical areas of our day-to-day life also can relieve—or cause—inflammation, depending on our approach. If you're fighting inflammation with food, you can use three more major weapons against inflammation at the same time: exercise, sleep, and stress management. The math is pretty simple here (aside from four weapons are better than one): If you get poor sleep, don't exercise, and are always stressed out, you're inflammation levels will no doubt be higher. If you're physically active, respect sleep, and manage your stress levels, your inflammation will most likely be lower. For all the details on how and why this works, see the special three-part section at the end of the book. All of these things tie together and can complement one another.

But it's even bigger than that, especially when you consider your mindset and how you approach lifestyle. If you're able to follow this eating plan for two weeks and have positive results, you'll look better, feel better—all the things you'd expect. You'll be like, *I did it!* It would be easy for someone to say, "Hey, that's great but if you really want to live right, you should be exercising and sleeping better and reducing your stress load." Mostly because it's easy for people to say such things without thinking about what it takes to pull off. But in this case, sleep, stress, and exercise all have positive or negative effects on inflammation, depending on which way you go. If you set your mind to work on all four aspects—legs on a table, so to speak—your whole mindset can change. You'll see what's possible. Better still, you'll see what's possible *for you*. You can go from *I can do this* to *I will do this* to *I did this,* and it won't be about just food, but your entire way of living. That's powerful. One good change feeds more good changes. For two weeks, you can commit to one thing—eating—and that's fine. Or you can commit to one big thing—a holistic lifestyle that can change your health.

Imagine how good achieving that will feel every day as you go. All you have to do is set your mind to it.

MINDSET, STEP 7

Prepare for Day 14.

Two weeks go fast. That's why you need to think about that last day, Day 14. You'll soon be seeing the results of your 14-day commitment. Which brings a big question: Now what?

On one hand: You've learned amazing things, ate amazing meals, lived a lighter life, lost weight, improved your health. What comes next?

On the other hand: You've done all those things, but it's still very easy to look behind you and see your old life and habits. What comes next?

To answer a question with a question, ask yourself... *Who do I want to be?* You can be the new you or the old you. People have a hard time with this question. That's why you hear about so many people who successfully lost weight on a given diet plan and soon put all the weight back on and then some. Do you want to be that person? If so, well, it's easy. If not? Well, that can be easy, too, if you let it be. It's not hard at all to just keep going, to let the Anti-Inflammatory Diet become the anti-inflammatory lifestyle.

Remember, you're the hero of your story. It's your call to make. But here's a little hint: Whenever you're having doubts, return to this chapter and hit reset on the ol' mindset. It's that simple.

6

Your 14-Day Anti-Inflammatory Eating Plan

What to eat for the next two weeks to lose weight and feel great

WHEN STARTING a healthy eating program, some people like suggestions for exactly what to eat and when. If that's you, this 14-day meal plan on the following pages will start you off on the right track. Everything you need is right here. On the other hand, you can also use this chapter as a general guide and mix-n-match your own recipe ideas with the collections in Chapters 7 and 8.

Some helpful notes before following this plan:

On Counting Calories

Counting calories and grams of carbohydrates, protein,

fat, and fiber is unpleasant. It can turn mealtime into math homework, which is why it's such a turnoff for so many people. Now, in this book, most of the recipes in chapters 7 and 8 include calorie and nutrition numbers. In general, no recipe delivers more than 500 calories per serving. Smoothies and snacks come in at fewer than 300 calories.

If you're a die-hard calorie counter, by all means enjoy your math. But you can do just fine on this plan without breaking out the food scale and calculator. It comes down to your preference and which approach will help you be successful.

On Total Calories

Based on the meal plan layout you're about to read, your daily food intake comes down to breakfast, a morning snack or "Smoothie of the Day," lunch, afternoon snack, and dinner. Total daily calorie counts vary, but generally speaking, you'll be consuming about 1,500 calories per day. You will lose weight on that moderately low-calorie diet. Remember, also, that you're changing the content of your diet and packing far more nutrients into those 1,500 calories. The quality improves as the quantity decreases.

Men, depending on their size, may require a few hundred more calories per day. You can easily adjust by taking a slightly larger portion size, or adding a little more protein and more vegetables, whole grains, or fruit. Or perhaps an evening snack. You've got flexibility here.

Man or woman, if you still feel hungry after a meal, have a second glass of water and wait five or 10 minutes. Usually hunger will subside. If still hungry, have some more vegetables to fill up. The goal is to learn to listen to your body's hunger cues and make adjustments according to

Why Eight is Great

Strive to drink your eight glasses of water daily. Why? Drinking lots of water during the day can make it easier to lose weight. For one, thirst is often misunderstood for hunger. Try answering a hunger pang with a zero-calorie glass of water and see how you feel five minutes later. The amount of water you drink may also impact your blood sugar levels. Not long ago, a study of 3,615 men and women conducted by the French National Research Institute found that people who drink very little water, a few glasses each day, may be more likely to develop abnormally high blood sugar. While monitoring 700 of these study participants over nine years, the researchers found that people who drank 17 ounces of water or more per day were 28 percent less likely to develop high blood sugar than those who drank less. Why? One possibility: If you're drinking water all day, you're not drinking calorie-laden drinks like soda and juice that contain added sugar. There could be another factor at play: *vasopressin*. This hormone acts as an anti-diuretic to help regulate water retention in the body. When you become dehydrated, vasopressin is produced to signal the kidneys to conserve water, which may elevate blood sugar.

To drink more water each day, keep a tumbler full of ice water with you at your desk at work and take it wherever you go. Sip constantly. And remember that you get a lot of water from the anti-inflammatory foods you eat, especially fresh vegetables and fruits.

---

your body's needs. Also, you have a life to lead. After you've eaten, move on, do what you need to do. Your day doesn't have to revolve around food. You simply need to eat three healthy meals and two snacks. As long as you're focusing on anti-inflammatory food combinations, you'll do fine.

On Being Prepared

It's easier to eat healthy when you have healthy food to eat. At the start of your 14-Day Anti-Inflammatory Diet, go food shopping to stock up on the ingredients you'll need to prepare healthy meals.

Tip: Start the plan on a Monday. The day before, prepare some snacks and meals for the week. Doing so will help you avoid rushing out for fast food when hunger strikes and healthy alternatives aren't available. If you plan ahead, however, healthy alternatives can *always* be available.

On Being Honest with Yourself

Yes, let's be honest. You know when you're doing certain things. Like sneaking unhealthy, inflammatory foods. Or overeating any foods. You know what added sugars do to your body. You know it's really, really hard to eat too many vegetables. So be honest with yourself about what, and how, you eat. You know you can play with this meal plan, add in your own versions of anti-inflammatory recipes, change when and what you'll eat, and what it takes to be successful. Just be honest with yourself about everything you do. That, perhaps more than anything, leads to success.

Instant Snacks

Simple. Convenient. Fast. And healthy! All of these quick ideas include anti-inflammatory foods and come in at 300 calories or less. Oh, and you might notice that there are 14 suggestions here. Fourteen days in the plan. Just sayin'...

- A piece of fruit (apples and oranges travel well)
- Handful of nuts
- Hardboiled egg dipped in brown mustard
- ½ cup DIY trail mix (nuts and dried fruit)
- ¼ cup hummus and vegetable slices for dipping
- ¼ cup guacamole and vegetable slices for dipping
- Banana with 1 tablespoon almond butter
- 2 whole grain crackers topped with 1 tablespoon tuna salad and grape tomato
- ½ cup Greek yogurt with berries and 1 tablespoon sliced almonds
- Half a banana dipped in 1 ounce melted dark chocolate
- Hard-boiled egg halves topped with 1 teaspoon guacamole and dash of hot sauce
- Sliced apple with 1 tablespoon almond butter
- ½ cup Greek yogurt with ½ cup sliced strawberries and 2 sliced kiwi fruit, 1 tablespoon sliced almonds
- ½ cup canned black beans, rinsed, mixed with fresh salsa to taste

For a heap of additional snack ideas, see the "Snackin' Sections," in Chapter 8!

14-DAY SAMPLE MEAL PLAN

Day 1

Breakfast: Strawberry Almond Overnight Oats (recipe p. 124)
Smoothie of the Day: Mexican Chocolate (recipe p. 118)
Lunch: Tuna-Guac Special (recipe p. 135)
Snack: Banana with 1 tablespoon of almond butter
Dinner: Chicken Spinach Parm (recipe p. 150)

Day 2

Breakfast: Leftover Quinoa Breakfast Bowl (recipe p. 126)
Smoothie of the Day: Bright & Blue (recipe p. 115)
Lunch: Quickie Quesadilla (recipe p. 131)
Snack: 2 whole grain crackers topped with 1 tablespoon tuna salad and grape tomato
Dinner: Pan Seared Halibut with Chickpeas, Cucumbers, and Cherry Tomatoes (recipe p. 147)

Day 3

Breakfast: Southwest Scramble (recipe p. 125)
Smoothie of the Day: Chocolate Peppermint Perfection (recipe p. 116)
Lunch: Grilled Vegetable Wrap (recipe p. 130)
Snack: ½ cup Greek yogurt with berries and 1 tablespoon sliced almonds
Dinner: Tuna Fish Lettuce Wraps with Strawberry Spinach Salad (recipe p. 145)

Day 4

Breakfast: Berry Best Oats (recipe p. 123)
Smoothie of the Day: DIY Detox (recipe p. 116)
Lunch: Smoked Salmon Sandwich (recipe p. 131)
Snack: ¼ cup guacamole and vegetable slices for dipping
Dinner: Chicks & Sticks Chopped Salad (recipe p. 143)

Day 5

Breakfast: Spicy Avocado Toast with Fried Egg and Tomato (recipe p. 124)
Smoothie of the Day: Unbeetable (recipe p. 120)
Lunch: English Muffin Pizzas (recipe p. 134)
Snack: Half a banana dipped in 1 ounce melted dark chocolate
Dinner: Taco Salad with Homemade Spices (recipe p. 146)

Day 6

Breakfast: Holy Guacamole Burrito (recipe p. 127)
Smoothie of the Day: Anti-Inflammatory Supersoaker (recipe p. 120)
Lunch: Turkey Noodle Soup with Spinach (recipe p. 134) and California Club Sandwich (recipe p. 135)
Snack: 1/4 cup hummus and vegetable slices for dipping
Dinner: Baked Salmon with Beets, Citrus, Avocado, and Caraway Seeds (recipe p. 144)

Day 7

Breakfast: Apple Almond Oatmeal (recipe p. 123)
Smoothie of the Day: Pear Punch (recipe p. 118)
Lunch: Chicken Fajita Burrito (recipe p. 132)
Snack: Hard-boiled egg halves topped with 1 teaspoon guacamole and dash of hot sauce
Dinner: Grilled Caesar Salad with Avocado Dressing (recipe p. 141)

Day 8

Breakfast: Banana Split (recipe p. 124)
Smoothie of the Day: Sweet Green (recipe p. 119)
Lunch: Roasted Butternut and Spinach Salad (recipe p. 138)
Snack: 1/2 cup DIY trail mix (nuts and dried fruit)
Dinner: Tandoori Chicken Thighs with Roasted Broccoli (recipe p. 142)

Day 9

Breakfast: Strawberry Almond Overnight Oats (recipe p. 124)
Smoothie of the Day: Tea Time (recipe p. 119)
Lunch: Tuna-Guac Special (recipe p. 135)
Snack: Sliced apple with 1 tablespoon almond butter
Dinner: Chicks & Sticks Chopped Salad (recipe p. 143)

Day 10

Breakfast: Banana Bread Mug Muffin (recipe p. 128)
Smoothie of the Day: Yummy-Healthy Chocolate Shake (recipe p. 120)
Lunch: Quickie Protein Salad (recipe p. 133)
Snack: Hard boiled egg dipped in brown mustard
Dinner: Hazelnut Crusted Salmon with Wilted Kale (recipe p. 142)

Day 11

Breakfast: Neat-o Burrito Bowl (recipe p. 126)
Smoothie of the Day: Berry Oatmeal in a Glass (recipe p. 115)
Lunch: Tabbouleh Salad with Quinoa (recipe p. 133)
Snack: ½ cup Greek yogurt with ½ cup sliced strawberries and 2 sliced kiwi fruit, 1 tablespoon sliced almonds
Dinner: Grilled Spicy Fish Tacos (recipe p. 148)

Day 12

Breakfast: Salmon Omelet (recipe p. 126)
Smoothie of the Day: Here Comes the Sun (recipe p. 116)
Lunch: PB&B Sandwich (recipe p. 136)
Snack: Handful of nuts
Dinner: Slimmed-Down Stuffed Peppers (recipe p. 149)

Day 13

Breakfast: Leftover Quinoa Breakfast Bowl (recipe p. 126)
Smoothie of the Day: Nut Butter Blast (recipe p. 118)
Lunch: Back-to-Your Roots Salad (recipe p. 137)
Snack: ½ cup canned black beans, rinsed, mixed with fresh salsa to taste
Dinner: Chicken Spinach Parm (recipe p. 150)

Day 14

Breakfast: Hearty Greek Egg Sandwich (recipe p. 128)
Smoothie of the Day: It's Easy Being Green (recipe p. 117)
Lunch: Avocado, Tomato, and Arugula Salad (recipe 136)
Snack: A piece of fruit (apple, pear, orange, etc)
Dinner: Tuna Fish Lettuce Wraps with Strawberry Spinach Salad (recipe p. 145)

7

A Smoothie a Day for 14 Days

Drink your way healthy and lean

OKAY, **DO YOU REALLY** have to have a smoothie a day on the 14-Day Anti-Inflammatory Diet? No. But why wouldn't you want to? Smoothies may be the most convenient food for someone trying to cut inflammation—and lose weight. Consider the following benefits:

They're easy to prepare. None of the recipes in this chapter take more than a few minutes. Your biggest chore will involve a knife and cutting board. And after a while, you won't have to measure; you'll be able to eyeball ingredient amounts.

They're packed with anti-inflammatory ingredients.
The most powerful anti-inflammatory foods happen to be fruits and vegetables. Which happen to be the primary ingredients in most smoothies. That means you also get tons of vitamins and fiber.

They're low calorie. Most recipes in this chapter have fewer than 300 calories a serving. Only one recipe in this chapter has more than 400. You can use them as meals or snacks.

They're versatile. You can make these recipes as is, or play around. Smoothie ingredients are only limited by your imagination. Stick to the anti-inflammatory foods from chapter 4 and you're golden.

They're easy to digest. The blender has taken a lot of the work out of it for your stomach (not to mention your jaw and teeth).

So let's take a look at smoothies. You'll find lots of ideas in this chapter, along with 15 simple and delicious anti-inflammatory recipes (one for each day, and one to grow on). First, here are some ideas on how to make smoothie-making easier and more convenient.

The Anti-Inflammatory Smoothie To-Do List

Pick a protein powder. A scoop or two of protein powder can add a terrific dose of muscle-building power and satiety to any smoothie—and some are packed with extra nutrients and flavors. But beware: Some powders are also infused with two things you *don't* want: unpronounceable chemicals and added sugar. Avoid! All that said, the big question is, for an anti-inflammatory diet, which protein should you choose? The more traditional whey protein powder preferred by fitness buffs or a vegetable-based powder? Or other options?

Whey protein has lots of nutritional benefits: It aids in muscle growth and recovery, may help control blood sugar spikes, and has been linked to prostate cancer prevention in some research. However, it's derived from dairy (a by-product of cheese production), and dairy has been shown to have inflammatory tendencies. Still, one study found that a protein in whey had an anti-inflammatory effect on the digestive systems of rats. And a whey protein called lactoferrin (found in high levels in breast milk) has been mentioned as a potential anti-inflammatory. Research is hardly conclusive, however. For this program, feel free to sub in whey protein, just know that it may work against your anti-inflammatory goals. And one last bit: A scoop of whey protein will add anywhere from 100 to 150 calories to your smoothie.

Plant protein powder is non-dairy and generally lactose- and gluten-free. You'll find powders derived from soy, brown rice, hemp, pea, beans, and even mixtures of those and more like quinoa, buckwheat, and flax. The calorie load is slightly lower than whey—100 calories a scoop or sometimes lower—and the anti-inflammatory benefits are in the mix because of the plant-based sourcing. One knock against vegetable proteins is that some types don't provide a complete chain of essential amino acids for building muscle. However, many brands combine different types of plant proteins to take care of that problem. See "Protein

Powders We Like" on page 112 for a list of our favorite protein powders.

Consider buying a new blender. Your old blender might be just fine. But it might not be strong enough for the job. You need something with enough horsepower to break up ice cubes or chunks of frozen berries and turn vegetables into drinkable fiber. You'll be more likely to make daily smoothies with a machine that's a breeze to use and clean.

Stock up on produce. There's nothing like a smoothie made with fresh ingredients. So turn your kitchen into a wannabe farmer's market. Fresh produce isn't an option? No worries. Just...

Pack your freezer. Stock up on frozen fruits and vegetables even if you have access to fresh. That way you'll always have options in a pinch. Your grocery store's frozen section is literally packed with flash-frozen produce that's just brimming with nutrients and waiting to jump into your blender. Quick tip: Many recipes ask for a banana—one of the most common natural ways to sweeten up a smoothie. Just buy a bunch, let them get reasonably ripe, then slice them into chunks and spread them on a wax-paper-covered baking pan. Stow it in the freezer for an hour, then put the frozen chunks in a zip-top bag, and you have a perfect go-to ingredient that won't spoil.

Stock up on nut milks. They're the perfect liquid base for a smoothie, particularly almond milk. Try different flavors for variety—vanilla and chocolate are always welcome—but whenever possible, go for unsweetened.

CRAZY IDEA OF THE DAY:
Add Algae to Your Smoothie

Spirulina is a high-protein seaweed supplement that's typically dried and sold in powdered form. The dried stuff is about 60 percent protein, and, like quinoa, it's a complete protein—deeming it a great weight loss tool. A tablespoon of the blue-green algae delivers 8 grams of metabolism-boosting protein for just 43 calories, plus half a day's allotment of vitamin B12, which can encourage weight loss by giving you more energy and boosting your metabolism. Experiment with spirulina in your smoothies and get a protein boost.

Add water if any concoction is too thick. Also, a few ice cubes will cool it down and make it more like a milkshake.

Remember, everything's optional. Some ingredients in these recipes are listed as optional, but the fact is, up to this point you've read a lot about the kinds of foods that battle inflammation. So feel free to experiment with these concoctions. For example, think about oats. Some good old fashioned rolled oats are a great smoothie ingredient because if you blend everything until smooth, they generally dissolve, so you get the goodness of oatmeal without having to fire up the stovetop. And play around with fruits by the season: Summer brings berries and nectarines. Autumn is great for pears and apples.

Enjoy! The recipes starting on page 115 are designed to fight inflammation, but the first order of business is "be delicious."

Protein Powders We Like

Eat This, Not That! tested an array of protein powders—including vegetable-based powders—that bring extra nutrition, anti-inflammatory power, and blender-friendly smoothness. All are readily available at online retailers and health food outlets.

Plant-Based Proteins:

Garden of Life Raw Meal. This organic protein blend is derived from belly-blasting brown rice, quinoa, and beans, plus tea and cinnamon extract—all proven inflammation fighters. With 20 grams of protein and 7 grams of fiber per serving with a reasonable 120 calories, having one of these for lunch before a workout will keep you feeling full and energized while preserving muscle. **$37.99.**

Jarrow Brown Rice. Another vegan-friendly option, Jarrow's Brown Rice Protein Concentrate has a surprisingly few amount of carbs (3 grams) and 0 grams of sugar per serving, so it's an excellent option for people looking to lose weight. With just 11 grams of protein, however, it might need to be supplemented with more protein-rich ingredients: raw almonds, nut butters, or plain lowfat Greek yogurt. The vanilla flavor makes a tasty base for bananas and berries, or blended with almond butter, cocoa powder, and unsweetened vanilla almond milk for a more decadent-tasting treat. **$9.36.**

Nutiva Organic Hemp. This protein powder won't give you the munchies—on the contrary, it will curb those junk food cravings—and you don't even need a license to enjoy it. Hemp protein (made with the less-fun parts of the plant) offers not only a decent amount of protein at 15 grams a serving, but also a healthy dose of fiber at 8 grams to keep you fuller, longer. With no artificial colors or ingredients and just 1 gram of natural sugar per serving, this powder is a clean option. But by itself, it isn't the most palatable. That's where smoothies come in; mix this powder with fresh fruit, your favorite leafy green, and some unsweetened almond milk for a rich, filling meal. **$11.95.**

Sun Warrior Blend Natural. Sun Warrior gets its protein from raw organic pea, cranberry, and hemp seed protein. And we love sticking with the natural flavor because it makes the best base for all your favorite smoothie fixin's; add in raw cocoa powder, a ripe banana, and unsweetened vanilla almond milk for a chocolaty taste, or keep it strictly fruity with a combo of berries, bananas, or tropical fruits. But if a more pronounced flavor is what you're looking for, Sun Warrior also comes in berry, chocolate, mocha, and vanilla. **$44.99.**

Vega One Natural. Vega One comes complete with six servings of greens, probiotics, antioxidants, and half your day's serving of vitamins and minerals, so it's pretty great all on its own with less than 1 gram of sugar and a whopping 20 grams of protein per serving. But throw in some nutrient-rich spinach, half a banana, and a handful of berries, and you have one of the cleanest, healthiest smoothies possible. Plus, its super smooth texture blends perfectly with your favorite ingredients without a gritty or chalky taste. The natural version makes a nice base for more veggie-packed smoothies, but opt for the delicious French Vanilla or Chocolate for a more dessert-like consistency. **$27.90.**

Animal-Based Proteins:

Naked Whey. The name says it all; the only ingredient in Naked Whey is whey protein concentrate from grass-fed cows. With 25 grams of protein per serving and just 3 grams of carbs, it's another great option for gym rats and those looking to drop a couple pounds. The unflavored version is as blank of a canvas as you can get for your favorite smoothie ingredients; it has a smooth, creamy texture that blends nicely with fruit, veggies, nut milks, and more. **$85.49 (for 5 lbs).**

Paleo Protein Egg White. Another animal-based protein powder, egg white protein is smart choice for people wanting to build lean muscle mass with 25 grams of protein a serving, and just 1 gram of sugar and 1 gram of carbs. It instantly dissolves in water and is completely flavorless, so it's the perfect base for more green-heavy smoothies and other lower-calorie options made with water instead of milk or yogurt. Since it doesn't leave a gritty texture, you'll barely realize it's even in your smoothie, except for the filling serving of protein. **$29.99.**

Source Organic Whey. Whey protein is one of the most popular forms of protein powders; the dairy derivative lines shelf after shelf in health food stores and supplement shops. That's because it's a complete protein, which means it contains all nine essential amino acids and will stimulate protein synthesis after a workout. Although it's a great option for fitness fanatics, the type and quality of whey varies drastically. If you can stomach whey (some dairy-sensitive people might not be able to), this non-GMO and organic option comes from grass-fed cows, delivering the highest nutrition of whey possible (with hopefully the least inflammation). With 21 grams of protein per serving and just 1 gram of naturally-occurring sugar, it doesn't need much dressing up in the form of a smoothie, but some fresh or frozen fruit and nut milk might make it go down easier. **$24.99.**

THE ANTI-INFLAMMATORY DIET SMOOTHIES

Here are the deviously simple instructions for making all these smoothie recipes: Combine ingredients in a blender. Blend until smooth. Drink!

Berry Oatmeal in a Glass

½ cup old fashioned rolled oats
1 cup low-fat milk or almond milk
½ cup frozen blueberries (any berries will do)
1 Tbsp honey (or to taste)
⅓ cup Greek yogurt
¼ cup ice

Makes 2 servings

Per serving: 220 calories, 5 g fat (2.3 g saturated), 32.75 g carbohydrates, 3.3 g fiber, 11 g protein

Bright & Blue

½ cup unsweetened almond milk
1 scoop vanilla protein powder
½ cup frozen blueberries
½ Tbsp unsalted almond butter
Water to blend (optional)

Makes 1 serving

Per serving: 232 calories, 6 g fat (0 g saturated), 16.5 g carbohydrates, 3 g fiber, 28 g protein

Chocolate Peppermint Perfection

1   frozen banana, sliced
2-3 ice cubes
1   cup unsweetened almond milk (chocolate almond milk works well)
1   scoop chocolate protein powder
2   Tbsp cocoa powder
Pinch of salt
¼   tsp peppermint extract
Several mint leaves (optional)

Makes 1 serving

Per serving: 153 calories, 3 g fat (1 g saturated), 18.5 g carbohydrates, 3 g fiber, 13 g protein

DIY Detox

1   cup unsweetened almond milk
1   frozen banana, sliced
½   cup frozen blueberries
2   tsp ginger, grated
2   cups kale
1   Tbsp chia seeds (optional)
Sprinkle of ground cinnamon
1-2 tsp honey (to taste)

Makes 1 serving

Per serving: 308 calories, 4 g fat (0.5 g saturated), 61 g carbohydrates, 8 g fiber, 7 g protein

Here Comes the Sun

4-6 oz Greek yogurt
1   cup frozen mixed berries
1   frozen banana, sliced
1   peeled and segmented orange

Makes 1 serving

Per serving: 209 calories, 1.8 g fat (0 g saturated), 40.2 g carbohydrates, 6 g fiber, 8 g protein

It's Easy Being Green

1	cup unsweetened almond milk
1	scoop vanilla protein powder
1	large handful of organic baby spinach
¼	cup frozen mango chunks
¼	cup frozen pineapple
½	banana (fresh or frozen)
1	Tbsp ground flax (optional)
1	Tbsp chia seeds (optional)

Makes 1 serving

Per serving: 231 calories, 8 g fat (0 g saturated), 21g carbohydrates, 9 g fiber, 19 g protein

Little Bit o' the Burn

½	cup unsweetened almond milk
1	cup chopped kale leaves
½	small cucumber, chopped
½	avocado, chopped
1	nectarine or peach, pitted and chopped (or 1 cup berries)
1	Tbsp lemon juice
½	- inch slice ginger, peeled and chopped
⅛	tsp cayenne pepper
10	ice cubes

Makes 2 servings

Per serving: 124 calories, 7 g fat (2 g saturated), 11.25 g carbohydrates, 5 g fiber, 4 g protein

Mexican Chocolate

1   cup unsweetened almond milk
3   ice cubes
½   frozen banana, sliced
4   Tbsp cocoa powder
1   tsp chili powder
1   tsp cinnamon
1   scoop chocolate protein powder
1   tsp flax seed oil (optional)

Makes 1 serving

Per serving: 290 calories, 11 g fat (9 g saturated), 27.75 g carbohydrates,
3 g fiber, 20 g protein

Nut Butter Blast

1   frozen banana, sliced
¾   cup unsweetened almond milk
1   Tbsp unsweetened almond butter
¼   cup old fashioned rolled oats
1   Tbsp chia seeds
Ground cinnamon
1   Tbsp raw cacao powder

Makes 1 serving

Per serving: 280 calories, 14 g fat (1 g saturated), 30.5 g carbohydrates,
9 g fiber, 8 g protein

Pear Punch

1   fresh or frozen pear, cut into small pieces
½   frozen banana, sliced
½   tsp cinnamon
½   cup low-fat milk or unsweetened almond milk
Handful of spinach (optional)

Makes 1 serving

Per serving: 332 calories, 14 g fat (3 g saturated), 45.5 g carbohydrates,
10 g fiber, 6 g protein

Sweet Green

¼   cup no-sugar-added apple juice
¼   cup water
½   scoop plant-based vanilla protein powder
½   fresh or frozen pear, chopped
½   cup baby spinach, loosely packed
½   frozen banana, sliced
¼   avocado

Makes 1 serving

Per serving: 271 calories, 6 g fat (0g saturated), 39 g carbohydrates,
8 g fiber, 15 g protein

Tea Time

½   cup unsweetened almond milk
½   cup chai tea (brewed from a teabag and chilled; any tea will do)
½   scoop plant-based vanilla protein powder
½   frozen banana, sliced
½   tsp ground cinnamon
½   Tbsp almond butter

Makes 1 serving

Per serving: 219 calories, 9 g fat (0g saturated),
17.5 g carbohydrates, 4 g fiber, 17 g protein

The Anti-Inflammatory Supersoaker

1 avocado, chopped
2 apples, cored and chopped (peels optional)
½ cup broccoli florets, chopped
1 small hunk ginger, peeled and grated (or finely chopped)
¼ cup parsley
Juice from ½ lime
2 leaves kale
1 cup brewed, cooled green tea (any will do)
⅔ cup unsweetened almond milk (or water)
2 tsp chia seeds (optional)

Makes 2 servings

Per serving: 365 calories, 21 g fat (4 g saturated), 39 g carbohydrates, 13 g fiber, 5 g protein

---

Unbeetable

½ cup unsweetened almond milk (or water)
1 cup fresh or frozen strawberries
1 frozen banana, sliced
1 medium beet, finely chopped
1 Tbsp honey, or to taste

Makes 2 servings

Per serving: 165 calories, 7.3 g fat (6 g saturated), 24 g carbohydrates, 4 g fiber, 2 g protein

---

Yummy-Healthy Chocolate Shake

½ cup unsweetened almond milk
1½ Tbsp raw cacao powder
1 Tbsp honey
1 frozen banana, sliced
2 Tbsp peanut butter (or any nut butter)

Makes 1 serving

Per serving: 437 calories, 19 g fat (4.4 g saturated), 54 g carbohydrates, 11 g fiber, 12.4 g protein

14-Day Anti-Inflammatory Diet Recipes

Healthy ideas for breakfast, lunch, dinner, and some serious snackin'

IF YOU'RE TRYING to make better food choices—or, say, maybe, perhaps revamping your entire way of eating for, say, maybe, perhaps a two-week period—your biggest allies aren't people, but ideas. Ideas give you options. Options offer variety. Variety means never getting bored with the same old meals. Chapter 4 was all about showing you what kind of foods help fight inflammation. This chapter is all about giving you delicious, easy-to-make recipes that employ all those foods.

Let's review a few things about what you'll see here—and what you won't. Anti-inflammatory foods are generally loaded with things like healthy fats, antioxidants, and fiber, which means a lot of fruits and vegetables. Does this mean your menu is meatless? No, but it can be if you want it to be. That's your choice. You'll find some lean proteins like poultry and fish options in here. What you won't find? Red meat (grass-fed beef can be a healthy option and feel free to add it to your diet, but keeping beef and processed meats out of these recipes is the easier option for people who want quick, uncomplicated eating suggestions). Added sugars. Refined flours. Food from a box.

Another helpful thought: Almost all of these recipes come in under 500 calories a serving. They're generally high in fiber and protein, so they're high-satiety, too. And as previously stated, each recipe is a generous combination of anti-inflammatory foods listed in Chapter 4. The stated goal: easy, filling, and healthy so you don't have to think about it. Now it's time for some recipes.

BREAKFAST IDEAS

There's some truth to the old adage that breakfast is the "most important meal of the day," and if you're looking to blast belly fat, what you eat at the start of each day can make all the difference. According to a study from the University of Missouri-Columbia, a high-fiber, high-protein breakfast may be the most important investment you can make for your waistline. The study showed that eating breakfast triggered people's brains to release dopamine, a feel-good chemical that helps to control impulses. In other words, eating a balanced breakfast decreases your chances of reaching for that 3 p.m. candy bar and keeps your belly slim.

The best part about these breakfast ideas? They're loaded with anti-inflammatory ingredients, of course, but you can prepare any of them in about 5 minutes.

Berry Best Oats

½   cup unsweetened almond milk
½   cup water
½   cup rolled oats
¼   tsp vanilla extract
¼   tsp ground cinnamon
¼   cup blueberries (fresh or frozen and thawed)
¼   cup blackberries (fresh or frozen and thawed)

Bring the almond milk and water to a boil. Stir in the oats and cook until soft, about 3 minutes. Just before the oats are finished, remove from the heat and stir in the vanilla and cinnamon, followed by the blueberries and blackberries.

Makes 1 serving

Per serving: 222 calories, 5 g fat (0 g saturated), 37 g carbohydrates, 7 g fiber, 10 g protein

Apple Almond Oatmeal

½   cup unsweetened almond milk
½   cup water
½   cup rolled oats
¼   tsp ground cinnamon
½   red apple, cored and chopped (skin on)
1   Tbsp raw flaked almonds

Bring the almond milk and water to a boil. Stir in the oats and cook until soft, about 3 minutes. Just before the oats are finished, remove from the heat and stir in the cinnamon, followed by the apple. Top with the almonds.

Makes 1 serving

Per serving: 244 calories, 8 g fat (0 g saturated), 37 g carbohydrates, 6 g fiber, 6 g protein

Spicy Avocado Toast with Fried Egg and Tomato

While a slice of whole grain bread toasts, fry an egg in a nonstick pan. Mash half an avocado directly on the toast, and sprinkle with paprika, salt, and pepper (or a dash of hot sauce). Layer on two slices of tomato and top with your egg.

Strawberry Almond Overnight Oats

⅛ cup rolled oats
2 Tbsp chia seeds
1 cup unsweetened almond milk
1 tsp vanilla extract
¼ cup strawberries, sliced
2 Tbsp sliced almonds

Mix the oats, chia seeds, almond milk, and vanilla. Refrigerate overnight. Serve topped with strawberries and almonds.

Makes 1 serving

Per serving: 341 calories, 19 g fat (2 g saturated), 28.5 g carbohydrates, 15 g fiber, 14 g protein

Breakfast Banana Split

½ cup unsweetened almond milk
½ cup water
½ cup rolled oats
1 Tbsp vanilla plant-based protein powder mixed with 1 Tbsp water until smooth (optional)
¼ banana, sliced
¼ cup strawberries, sliced (fresh or frozen and thawed)
1 Tbsp dark chocolate chips

Bring the almond milk and water to a boil. Stir in the oats and cook until soft, about 3 minutes. Just before the oats are finished, remove from the heat and stir in the protein powder, if using, followed by the banana and strawberries. Top with the chocolate chips.

Makes 1 serving

Per serving: 296 calories, 9 g fat (0 g saturated), 47 g carbohydrates, 6 g fiber, 11 g protein

---

Southwest Scramble

1   Tbsp extra-virgin olive oil
2   Tbsp minced onion
¼   cup diced red bell pepper
2   eggs
¼   cup black beans
¼   avocado, chopped
2   Tbsp cilantro

Heat the oil in a frying pan and add onion and bell pepper, stirring until softened. Add eggs, beans, avocado, and cilantro, and cook until the eggs are cooked to your preferred consistency.

Makes 1 serving

Per serving: 480 calories, 37.5 g fat (8 g saturated), 17 g carbohydrates, 8 g fiber, 18 g protein

---

A TASTY IDEA

Peaches and Cream Yogurt Parfait

Grate about a tablespoon of fresh ginger into a cup of plain yogurt with a tablespoon of honey, and stir to combine. Top with sliced peaches and flax seeds.

Neat-o Burrito Bowl

½   cup black beans
¼   cup store-bought pico de gallo or salsa
1   fried or poached egg
½   avocado, cubed

Layer the ingredients in a bowl, beans and avocado first, then the egg topped with pico de gallo.

Makes 1 serving

Per serving: 376 calories, 22 g fat (4 g saturated), 29.5 g carbohydrates, 15 g fiber, 15 g protein

---

Salmon Omelet

2   eggs, whisked
2   oz canned salmon, flaked
¼   avocado, cubed
½   cup baby arugula
1   Tbsp hemp seeds

Pour whisked eggs into an omelet pan on medium heat. As they cook, add salmon, avocado, and seeds. After a few minutes, fold eggs over to cover ingredients. Serve on bed of arugula.

Makes 1 serving

Per serving: 496 calories, 37 g fat (7 g saturated), 11g carbohydrates, 8 g fiber, 30 g protein

A TASTY IDEA
Leftover Quinoa Breakfast Bowl

In a bowl, combine cooked quinoa with a half-cup almond milk and pop it in the microwave to warm up, 1 to 2 minutes. Stir to mix and top with strawberries, pecans, and a drizzle of balsamic vinegar.

Holy Guacamole Burrito

2   eggs
1   medium whole-wheat tortilla
2   slices fat-free turkey deli slices
½   avocado, sliced
2   Tbsp shredded reduced-fat Mexican-blend cheese

Scramble the eggs in a skillet or the microwave. Then arrange all the ingredients on the tortilla, fold the ends, then neatly roll.

Makes 1 serving

Per serving: 349 calories, 22 g fat (5 g saturated),
19.75 g carbohydrates, 8 g fiber, 18 g protein

A TASTY IDEA
One-Pot Spicy Eggs

Simmer half a can of black beans with a cup of chicken stock. Crack two eggs directly into the mixture and cook until the whites are set. Hit it with plenty of hot sauce.

Hearty Greek Egg Sandwich

1   whole egg
1   egg white
1   toasted whole wheat English muffin
¼   cup baby spinach
¼   cup mashed avocado
1   Tbsp crumbled feta
2   tomato slices

Scramble 1 whole egg with 1 egg white in a skillet coated with cooking spray. Place on toasted whole wheat English muffin spread with ¼ cup mashed avocado, and top with 1 slice reduced-fat Cheddar cheese, tomato slices, and baby spinach.

Makes 1 serving

Per serving: 367 calories, 17 g fat (4 g saturated), 29.5 g carbohydrates, 8.6 g fiber, 24 g protein

A TASTY IDEA
Banana Bread Mug Muffin

Whisk together 2 tablespoons of almond milk, a teaspoon of honey, a pinch of salt, and an egg. Add a quarter-cup of oats and a mashed banana, then stir until combined. Pop in the microwave for 2 minutes, checking the mug after every 30 seconds and waiting 10 seconds before putting it back in.

The Snackin' Section

Snacks should be quick. Snacks should be easy peasy to make. And the best ones are also brimming with healthy nutrients like these:

Avocado Cracker

What You'll Need: Multigrain crackers, avocado, tomato, salt, pepper

Layer a multigrain cracker with sliced avocado. Option: add ¼-inch-thick slice of plum or romano tomato. Sprinkle with salt and pepper.

Hummus & Veggies Mason Jars

What You'll Need: Peppers, celery, carrots, hummus

Using a tiny jar for hummus is great for perfecting portion control. Simply divide up your portioned servings of hummus and dip fiber-rich vegetables into the protein-packed puree.

Spiced Nuts

What You'll Need: walnuts, almonds, peanuts, cashews, chili powder, black pepper, cayenne

Toss a combination of nuts—walnuts, almonds, peanuts, cashews—with chili powder, black pepper, and a pinch of cayenne. Roast in a 400°F oven for 10 minutes until warm and toasty.

LUNCH IDEAS

Lunch is kind of an orphan meal. Stuck right in the middle of the day, but generally eaten away from home, usually when you're alone, especially if you're at work or out and about getting life done. You're busy, but use this time to break your day into two parts. The problem a lot of people have? The wrong lunch choice results in a food coma, or a fast-food hangover, or the always-popular delayed 3-pm-sleep-spiral. Here's the good news: These selections are hearty and filling, yet light and full of nutrient-dense anti-inflammatory foods. They won't sit in your belly like a lead sinker and put you to sleep. They're also designed for portability so you can make them at home beforehand and take them on the road or to the office.

Grilled Vegetable Wrap

12   asparagus spears, woody ends removed
2   Portobello mushroom caps
1   red bell pepper, halved, seeds and stem removed
1   Tbsp olive oil
2   Tbsp olive oil mayonnaise
1   Tbsp balsamic vinegar
1   clove garlic, minced
4   large spinach or whole-wheat tortillas or wraps
2   cups arugula or baby greens
¾   cup crumbled goat or feta cheese
Salt and ground black pepper to taste

Roast the vegetables in the oil in a 450°F oven for 10 to 12 minutes. Slice the mushroom caps and pepper into thin strips. Add the mayonnaise, vinegar, and garlic to a small bowl and stir to combine. Heat the tortillas on the grill or wrap them together in damp paper towels and heat in the microwave for 30 seconds. Spread the mayo down the middle of each tortilla, then top with the greens and cheese. Divide the grilled vegetables among the tortillas, salt and pepper, then roll up tightly and slice each wrap in half.

Makes 4 servings

Per serving: 240 calories, 13 g fat (3.5 g saturated), 22.25 g carbohydrates, 4.5 g fiber, 8.5 g protein

---

Smoked Salmon Sandwich

8   slices of whole wheat or 9-grain bread, toasted
¼   cup whipped cream cheese
2   Tbsp capers, rinsed and chopped
½   red onion, thinly sliced
2   cups mixed baby greens
1   large tomato, sliced
Salt and ground black pepper to taste
8   oz smoked salmon

Spread 1 tablespoon of the cream cheese on each of four slices of toast. Top each with capers, onion, greens, and a slice or two of tomato. Lightly salt the tomato, then add as much pepper as you'd like (this sandwich cries out for a lot of it). Finish by draping a few slices of smoked salmon over the tomatoes and topping each with one of the remaining slices of toasted bread.

Makes 4 servings

Per serving: 280 calories, 10 g fat (3 g saturated), 29.5 g carbohydrates, 5 g fiber, 18 g protein

---

A TASTY IDEA
Quickie Quesadilla

Sprinkle diced red bell pepper, tomato, and fresh jalapeno one side of a whole grain tortilla. Add two tablespoons of black beans, a sprinkle of grated low-fat Mexican cheese, and fold over the other side of the tortilla. Microwave for about 20 seconds. Cut the semi-circle into slices after letting it cool.

Chicken Fajita Burrito

½   Tbsp canola oil
1   large onion, sliced
1   red bell pepper, sliced
1   poblano or green bell pepper, sliced
Salt and ground black pepper to taste
½   can (14-16 oz) black beans, drained and rinsed
¼   tsp cumin
Juice of 1 lime
Hot sauce
4   (10-inch) whole wheat tortillas
1   cup low-fat shredded jack cheese
2   cups shredded chicken
Salsa (salsa verde is especially good here)

Heat the oil in a large skillet over high heat. Add the onion and red and
poblano peppers and cook until browned, about 7 to 8 minutes. Season
with salt and black pepper. Combine the beans with the cumin in a
saucepan and warm. Add lime and a few shakes of hot sauce. Preheat
a griddle, cast-iron skillet, or large nonstick pan over medium heat.
Microwave the tortillas for 20 seconds, just enough so they're pliable.
Building one burrito at a time, sprinkle on cheese, then top with beans,
onion-pepper mixture, chicken, and salsa. Roll into a tight package. Place
the burritos directly on the skillet, cooking for a minute on each side until
lightly toasted.

Makes 4 servings

Per serving: 340 calories, 12 g fat (6 g saturated), 36 g carbohydrates,
4 g fiber, 22 g protein

Quickie Protein Salad

1	5-ounce can tuna, drained
2	hard-cooked eggs, peeled and chopped
1	small carrot, shredded
¼	cup organic mayonnaise
1	Tbsp balsamic vinegar
½-1	tsp curry powder
2	large tomatoes (heirloom if available)

Grains of paradise or cracked black pepper

In a medium bowl stir together tuna, eggs, carrot, mayonnaise, vinegar, and curry powder. Core tomatoes. Cut each into wedges almost to but not through bottoms. Fan out wedges and top with tuna-egg salad. Season to taste with grains of paradise.

TIP:

* Read the labels when shopping for mayonnaise and opt for one with no added sugar, if possible. You can also make this with all or part Greek yogurt.

Makes 2 servings

Per serving: 431 calories, 32 g fat (7 g saturated), 11.75 g carbohydrates, 3 g fiber, 24 g protein

A TASTY IDEA
Tabbouleh Salad with Quinoa

Mix three-quarters of a cup of cooked quinoa in a bowl with diced cherry tomatoes, green onion, chopped cucumber, salt, and pepper. Toss it in a mixture of extra virgin olive oil and lemon juice. Add in chopped mint for extra flavor.

Turkey Noodle Soup with Spinach

4   oz whole wheat noodles, cooked
1   Tbsp canola oil
½   cup chopped onion
½   cup chopped carrot
½   cup chopped celery
1   tsp dried sage
12   oz ground turkey breast
2   cans (14 ½ ounces each) fat-free reduced-sodium chicken broth
4   cups water
1   Tbsp balsamic vinegar
½   tsp salt
1   bag (6 oz) baby spinach leaves
Ground black pepper

Cook the noodles according to the package directions. Drain and set aside. Meanwhile, in a pot over medium heat, warm the oil. Add the onion, carrot, celery, and sage. Cook, stirring occasionally, for 5 minutes, or until the vegetables start to soften. Add the turkey. Cook, breaking up the turkey with the back of a spoon, for about 4 minutes longer, or until the turkey is no longer pink. Add the broth, water, vinegar, and salt. Simmer for about 5 minutes, or until hot. Do not boil. Stir in the spinach and reserved noodles. Remove from the heat and let rest for 5 minutes. Season with pepper to taste.

Makes 8 servings

Per serving: 135 calories, 3 g fat (0.1 g saturated), 13 g carbohydrates, 2 g fiber, 14 g protein

A TASTY IDEA
English Muffin Pizzas

Preheat oven to 450°F. Top whole-wheat English muffin halves with marinara sauce, a sprinkle of cheese, and as many vegetables as you like (we use spinach, green peppers, broccoli, olives, and tomatoes). This will cook in roughly 3 minutes so be sure to keep an eye on the oven to prevent the cheese from burning.

California Club Sandwich

4   slices multigrain bread
1 ½ tsp Dijon mustard
½   cup thinly sliced cucumber
½   medium avocado, sliced, about 3 oz
½   jarred roasted red pepper, drained and halved
1 oz soft goat cheese, crumbled
¼   cup alfalfa sprouts

Place 2 slices of the bread on a work surface. Spread one side of each with the mustard. Top each with ¼ cup cucumber, one-half of the avocado, one-half of the roasted pepper, ½ ounce goat cheese, 2 tablespoons of the sprouts, and 1 of the remaining bread slices. Cut each in half.

Makes 2 servings

Per serving: 200 calories, 9 g fat (3 g saturated), 21.75 g carbohydrates, 8 g fiber, 8 g protein

Tuna-Guac Special

1   can chunk light tuna, drained
⅓ fresh avocado
Salt and pepper to taste (salt in tuna may be enough for some)
2   slices whole grain bread
Lettuce (optional)
Tomato (optional)
Onion (optional)

Mix tuna, avocado, salt and pepper. Spread on bread. Add lettuce, tomato, and onion if you like.

Makes 1 serving

Per serving: 375 calories, 10 g fat (1.7 g saturated), 28.25 g carbohydrates, 7 g fiber, 43 g protein

PB & B Sandwich

1   toasted whole wheat high-fiber English muffin
2   Tbsp peanut butter
¼   cup sliced banana
20   blueberries

Spread each half of a toasted whole wheat English muffin with 1
tablespoon peanut butter and top each half with 1/4 cup sliced banana.
Eat as an open-faced sandwich with a side of 20 blueberries

Makes 1 serving

Per serving: 405 calories, 18 g fat (3.7 g saturated),
45.75 g carbohydrates, 9 g fiber, 15 g protein

Avocado, Tomato, and Arugula Salad

2   Tbsp extra virgin olive oil
1   Tbsp balsamic vinegar
1   small clove garlic, crushed through a press
¼   tsp salt
¼   tsp ground black pepper
4   cups baby arugula
4   ripe medium tomatoes (about 12 oz total), cored and cut into
     wedges
1   large ripe avocado, halved, pitted, peeled, quartered, and sliced
     crosswise
¼   cup thinly sliced red onion
1   tsp toasted sunflower seeds (substitute with slivered almonds or
     pumpkin seeds)

In a salad bowl, whisk the oil, vinegar, garlic, salt, and pepper together.
Add the arugula, tomatoes, avocado, and onion; toss gently to mix.
Sprinkle with the sunflower seeds.

Makes 4 servings

Per serving: 217 calories, 7 g fat (1 g saturated), 30.5 g carbohydrates,
9 g fiber, 8 g protein

Back-To-Your-Roots Salad

1   15-oz can diced beets, drained
1   small jicama, peeled and cut into thin strips or diced
2   medium-size carrots, peeled and cut into thin strips or diced
3   Tbsp lemon juice
2   Tbsp seasoned rice vinegar
2   tsp stone-ground mustard
½   tsp dried dill weed

Place beet cubes in a large salad bowl, along with jicama and carrot pieces. In a small bowl mix lemon juice, vinegar, mustard, and dill; pour over the salad. Toss to mix. Serve warm or chilled.

Makes 6 servings

Per serving: 64 calories, 0.2 g fat (0 g saturated), 13.5 g carbohydrates, 6 g fiber, 2 g protein

Mexican Corn Salad

1   15-oz can corn, drained
1   large cucumber, peeled and diced
½   cup fine-chopped red onion
1   medium-size red bell pepper, diced fine
1   medium-size tomato, seeded and diced
½   cup chopped fresh cilantro (optional)
2   Tbsp seasoned rice vinegar
2   Tbsp apple cider or distilled vinegar
1   Tbsp lemon juice
1   clove garlic, minced
1   tsp ground coriander
⅛   tsp cayenne pepper

In a large salad bowl combine corn, cucumber, onion, pepper, tomato, and cilantro. In a small bowl combine vinegars, lemon juice, garlic, cumin, coriander, and cayenne. Pour over the salad and toss gently to mix.

Makes 6 servings

Per serving: 82 calories, 1 g fat (0 g saturated), 15.25 g carbohydrates, 3 g fiber, 3 g protein

Roasted Butternut and Spinach Salad

¾ lb precut butternut squash cubes (¾-inch) or ½ medium butternut
    squash, peeled, seeded, and cubed (2 cups)
1   large red bell pepper, cut into ¾-inch pieces
2   Tbsp extra virgin olive oil, divided
1   tsp chopped fresh thyme or ½ tsp dried thyme
½   tsp salt, divided
¼   tsp freshly ground black pepper, divided
2   Tbsp freshly squeezed lemon juice (about 1 lemon)
2   tsp honey
¼   small red onion, chopped, about ¼ cup
4   cups loosely packed baby spinach, 4 oz
1   small Gala or Golden Delicious apple, cored and thinly sliced
1   cup thinly sliced radicchio
½   cup unsalted sunflower seeds

Preheat oven to 425°F. Coat rimmed baking sheet with olive oil spray.
Toss squash and bell pepper with 2 teaspoons of the oil, thyme, ¼
teaspoon of the salt, and ⅛ teaspoon of the black pepper in medium
bowl. Arrange in single layer on prepared baking sheet. Roast 25 to 30
minutes, stirring occasionally to prevent sticking, until tender and lightly
browned. Let cool 10 minutes. Whisk lemon juice, honey, and remaining
4 teaspoons oil, ¼ teaspoon salt, and ¼teaspoon black pepper in
large salad bowl while squash roasts. Stir in onion. Add spinach, apple,
radicchio, sunflower seeds, and squash mixture and toss to combine.

Makes 4 servings

Per serving: 44 calories, 15 g fat (2 g saturated), 22.25 g carbohydrates,
7 g fiber, 5 g protein

Super-Healthy Fruit Salad

SWEET LIME DRESSING:

1   cup plain yogurt
½   cup red raspberries
¼   cup fresh lime juice
4   Tbsp honey
1   tsp vanilla extract

FRUIT SALAD:

2   peaches or nectarines, sliced
1   cup green or red grapes
1   cup honeydew chunks
1   cup pineapple chunks
1   cup red raspberries
1   cup blackberries
Mint leaves, for garnish

To make the sweet lime dressing: Place the yogurt, raspberries, lime juice, honey, and vanilla extract in a blender. Blend until smooth. To make the fruit salad: In a large bowl, combine the peaches, grapes, honeydew, pineapple, raspberries, and blackberries. Add the dressing and toss well. Allow to sit for 30 minutes, covered, at room temperature. Garnish with mint leaves just before serving.

ALTERNATE: Substitute other fruits as they're in season. Try strawberries, kiwi, cantaloupe, watermelon, papaya, or apricots. In the winter, use apples and pears, and top with a sprinkling of pomegranate seeds.

Makes 6 servings

Per serving: 151 calories, 0.6 g fat, 21 g carbohydrates, 5 g fiber, 3.4 g protein

The Snackin' Section

Need some snack ideas to take to work to curb those midday cravings? Try these suggestions that provide hunger satisfying fats, protein, and fiber:

D.I.Y. Trail Mix

What You'll Need: almonds, walnuts, cashew, sunflower seeds, dried fruit

Make your own suped-up trail mix: Combine 1 cup almonds, walnuts, or cashews (or a mix of all three) with ½ cup sunflower seeds and 1 ½ cups dried fruit: raisins, apricots, apples, prunes, and/or banana chips. Separate into small snack bags for portable snacking.

Berry Yogurt Toast

What You'll Need: Ezekiel toast, Greek yogurt, berries, chia seeds

Top a piece of fiber-rich Ezekiel toast with Greek yogurt and a variety of berries. Then sprinkle with chia seeds.

Corn & Bean Salsa with Chips

What You'll Need: Cooked corn, black beans, tomato, bell pepper, red onion, apple cider vinegar, lime juice, salt, and pepper. Tortilla chips are optional.

A perfect blend of corn, black beans, chopped tomatoes, chopped bell peppers, red onion, and dressed with a splash of apple cider vinegar and lime juice. Salt and pepper to taste. Serve either with chips or eat with a spoon (also works as a healthy side).

DINNER IDEAS

What better way to close out the day—especially a day of good food choices that have you feelin', well, pretty good—than with an easy-prep, relaxing sit-down with a plate of food you know is doing your body a solid. None of these entrees break the calorie bank and, like all the recipes in this chapter, are loaded with bonafide anti-inflammatory foods that also taste great.

Grilled Caesar Salad with Avocado Dressing

½   small avocado
¼   cup plain Greek yogurt
1   Tbsp apple cider vinegar
½   tsp Dijon-style mustard
1   tsp chopped fresh tarragon or chives
1   romaine heart, halved lengthwise
½   tsp olive oil
1   cup chopped cooked turkey, chicken, or canned tuna
1   slice sprouted bread, toasted and cubed for croutons

For the dressing, combine avocado, Greek yogurt, vinegar, mustard, and tarragon in a food processor bowl. Thin with water if needed until just pourable. Brush romaine halves with olive oil and grill, cut-sides down, for 4 to 6 minutes or until slightly charred on the edges. Transfer to two dinner plates. Spoon dressing over romaine; top with turkey and bread croutons.

Makes 2 servings

Per serving: 275 calories, 11 g fat (3 g saturated), 14 g carbohydrates, 5 g fiber, 30 g protein (calculated with 1 cup chopped turkey)

Hazelnut-Crusted Salmon with Wilted Kale

2   6-oz salmon fillets or arctic char fillets, skinned (3/4-inch thick)
2   Tbsp chopped hazelnuts, pecans, or raw pumpkin seeds
2   Tbsp coconut oil or butter, softened
2   Tbsp whole-wheat panko bread crumbs
1   Tbsp chopped chives or tarragon
2   tsp grated Pecorino or Parmesan cheese
¼   tsp garlic pepper

Preheat oven to 450°F. Place fish on one end of a foil-lined 15x10-inch baking pan. Stir together nuts, coconut oil, bread crumbs, herb, cheese, and lemon pepper. Spoon nut mixture onto fish and pat gently to spread. Bake fish for 6 to 8 minutes or until fish flakes with a fork. If desired, serve over Wilted Kale.

WILTED KALE: Toss 4 cups baby kale with 2 teaspoons olive oil and ¼ teaspoon salt. Place on the foil-lined baking pan next to the fish and bake for 3 to 4 minutes or just until wilted, tossing gently half way through baking time. If desired, drizzle with 2 teaspoons lemon juice.

Makes 2 servings.

Per serving: 432 calories, 25 g fat (14 g saturated), 10.75 g carbohydrates, 3 g fiber, 41 g protein

Tandoori Chicken Thighs with Roasted Broccoli

1   8-oz carton plain yogurt or plain coconut yogurt
1   Tbsp lemon juice
1   Tbsp garam masala seasoning
1   Tbsp grated ginger
½   tsp garlic salt
8   small bone-in chicken thighs, skinned

In a bowl combine yogurt, lemon juice, garam masala, ginger, and garlic salt. Place chicken in a 2-quart rectangular baking dish. Pour marinade over chicken. Cover and chill for 2 to 24 hours.

Preheat oven to 400°F. Place chicken on a rack in a shallow baking pan. Roast, uncovered, for 40 to 45 minutes or until no longer pink inside.

ROASTED BROCCOLI: Cut 1 head broccoli into florets, discarding woody stems. In a large bowl toss broccoli with 2 tablespoons olive oil and salt and lemon pepper to taste. Arrange on a foil-lined 15x10-inch baking pan and roast in the same oven as the chicken until crisp-tender and lightly browned on the edges (about 20 minutes).

Makes 4 servings

Per serving: 360 calories, 12 g fat (2 g saturated), 6 g carbohydrates, 1 g fiber, 57 g protein

---

Chicks & Sticks Chopped Salad

1	lemon
3	Tbsp olive oil
1	tsp Dijon-style or whole-grain mustard
1	9-oz bag romaine or a crunchy lettuce blend, coarsely chopped
1	15-oz can garbanzo beans (chickpeas), drained and rinsed
2	cups shredded cooked chicken*
3	cups matchstick vegetables (such as sweet peppers, carrots, cucumber, radish, green onions, and/or zucchini cut into matchstick-size strips or chopped)
¼	cup chopped dried tomatoes (oil pack), drained, or quartered Kalamata olives

Zest and juice the lemon. In a jar with a lid combine lemon juice, ½ teaspoon of the lemon zest, oil, and mustard. Cover and shake. In a large bowl layer lettuce, beans, chicken, matchstick vegetables, and tomatoes. Toss with dressing.

TIP:
* Leftover cooked skinless chicken or rotisserie chicken, shredded with two forks, works well.

Makes 4 servings

Per serving: 282 calories, 18 g fat (3 g saturated), 6 g carbohydrates, 3 g fiber, 24 g protein

Baked Salmon with Beets, Citrus, Avocado, and Caraway Seeds

4   5-oz portions of fresh wild salmon
4   large store-bought pre-roasted beets (not canned), cut into bite-size pieces
3   large oranges, segmented
1   Ruby Red grapefruit, segmented
1   cup chopped parsley
1   Tbsp caraway seeds, toasted in a dry pan over medium heat until fragrant (about 2 minutes)
½   avocado, diced
2   Tbsp vinaigrette dressing
Salt and pepper
2   Tbsp raw walnuts, toasted in a dry pan over medium heat until fragrant (about 2 minutes), and roughly chopped

Preheat the oven to 350°F. Season the fish with a pinch of salt and black pepper. Place on a non-stick sheet pan, skin side up, and place in the oven. Cook for 6 to 8 minutes. While the salmon is cooking, place the beets, whole orange and grapefruit segments, parsley, toasted caraway seed, avocado, and vinaigrette in a medium bowl and season with a pinch of salt and pepper. Mix well. Divide the salad among four plates, and top with the cooked salmon. Garnish with toasted walnuts.

Makes 4 servings

Per serving: 428 calories, 20 g fat (0 g saturated), 29 g carbohydrates, 8 g fiber, 33 g protein

Tuna Fish Lettuce Wraps with Strawberry Spinach Salad

TUNA WRAPS

1   lb canned light chunk tuna, drained
¼   cup mayonnaise
½   avocado, diced
2   hard-boiled eggs, diced
½   medium red onion, sliced thin
Salt and pepper
12   Bibb lettuce leaves (about 1 head)

SALAD

2   cups packed baby spinach
1   cup strawberries, quartered
2   Tbsp vinaigrette
2   Tbsp raw walnuts, toasted in a dry pan over medium heat until fragrant (about 2 minutes), and roughly chopped

Place the tuna in a medium size bowl, and use a spatula to fold in the mayonnaise, taking care not to break up the tuna too much. Gently fold in the avocado, hard boiled eggs, onion, and a pinch of salt and black pepper to taste. Place a spoonful of the tuna into a Bibb lettuce leaf and place on a plate. Repeat with the remaining tuna mixture and lettuce leaves, about 12 wraps total. Combine all the salad ingredients in a bowl and mix well. Divide the salad among four plates. Serve with three lettuce wraps.

Makes 4 servings

Per serving: 304 calories, 15 g fat (0 g saturated), 18.25 g carbohydrates, 6 g fiber, 24 g protein

Taco Salad with Homemade Spices

OLIVE OIL SPRAY

1   lb extra lean ground poultry
2   Tbsp Mexican Spice Blend (see below)
1   head iceberg lettuce, chopped into 1-inch cubes
1   cup salsa
½   cup guacamole

FOR THE MEXICAN SPICE BLEND:

2½   Tbsp chili powder
1   tsp kosher salt
4   tsp paprika
2   tsp ground cumin
4   tsp onion powder
4   tsp garlic powder

Mix spices in a glass bowl. Store in a BPA-free container out of direct sunlight for up to a month. Heat a large skillet sprayed with olive oil over medium high heat, and add the ground poultry. Use a rubber spatula or a wooden spoon to break up the ground poultry into small pieces until browned. Add the Mexican Spice Blend to the pan and mix well. Turn off heat, and use a slotted spoon to transfer the meat to a plate covered in paper towels to drain any excess fat. Divide the chopped iceberg lettuce among four plates, and top each salad with ¼ of the spicy meat. Top with ¼ cup salsa and 2 tablespoons guacamole.

Makes 4 servings

Per serving: 312 calories, 17 g fat (0 g saturated), 14.75 g carbohydrates, 5 g fiber, 25 g protein

Pan Seared Halibut with Chickpeas, Cucumbers, and Cherry Tomatoes

4   5-oz portions of halibut
Salt and pepper
1   Tbsp extra virgin olive oil
1   cup canned chickpeas, drained and rinsed
1   English cucumber, halved and sliced in half moons
1   cup cherry tomatoes, halved
½   avocado, diced into ¼-inch cubes
1   red pepper, diced into ¼-inch cubes
2   sprigs mint, coarsely chopped
¼   cup chopped parsley
¼   cup Kalamata olives, pits removed, halved
2   tsp whole cumin seed, toasted in a dry pan over medium heat until
    fragrant (about 2 minutes)
2   cups fresh baby spinach, packed 2 vinaigrette
Salt and pepper

Season the halibut with a pinch of salt and fresh ground pepper on both sides. Heat a nonstick pan over a medium heat, and add 1 tablespoon of olive oil. Add halibut to the pan, and cook until the fish starts to turn brown, about 3 minutes. Flip the fish over, and cook for an additional 5 minutes, or until the fish is firm to the touch. While the fish is cooking, place all the ingredients for the salad in a large bowl, season with a pinch of salt and pepper, and mix well. Divide the salad among four plates, and top with the warm halibut.

Makes 4 servings

Per serving: 375 calories, 17 g fat (0 g saturated), 20.5 g carbohydrates, 6 g fiber, 35 g protein

Grilled Spicy Fish Tacos

1   cup finely shredded red cabbage
12   oz mahi-mahi
2   limes
½   medium red onion, diced
4   corn tortillas
1   Tbsp Canola oil
1   mango, peeled, pitted, and cubed
1   avocado, peeled, pitted, and cubed
1   handful cilantro, chopped
Salt and pepper
½   Tbsp blackening spice

Clean and oil a grill or grill pan thoroughly. Preheat to medium-high.
Make the mango salsa by combining the mango, avocado, red onion,
cilantro, and the juice of one lime. Season to taste with salt and pepper.
Drizzle a light coating of oil over the fish, and rub on the blackening
spice. Place the fish on the grill and cook, undisturbed, for 4 minutes.
Carefully flip with a spatula and cook for another 4 minutes. Remove.
Before turning off the grill, warm the tortillas directly on the surface for 1
to 2 minutes. Divide the fish evenly among the warm tortillas, add a bit
of cabbage, and spoon the salsa on top. Serve each taco with a wedge of
lime and ½ cup of black beans spiked with cumin.

Makes 2 servings

Per serving: 610 calories, 18 g fat (3 g saturated), 56.5 g carbohydrates,
20g fiber, 45g protein

Slimmed-Down Stuffed Peppers

⅓   cup slivered almonds
1 ½ cups water
¼   tsp salt
¾   cup quinoa
4   large red, green, or yellow bell peppers
1   tsp olive oil
1   medium onion, chopped
2   large cloves garlic, minced

1   package (10 oz) fresh spinach, tough stems removed, torn into large
    pieces
½   cup crumbled feta cheese
¼   cup dried currants or raisins
1   can (14 ½ ounces) diced tomatoes
2   Tbsp tomato paste
¼   tsp dried Italian seasoning

Preheat the oven to 375°F. Cook the slivered almonds in a small nonstick
skillet over medium heat, stirring often, for 3 to 4 minutes, or until lightly
toasted. Tip onto a plate and let cool. In a saucepan, bring the water and
salt to a boil. Place the quinoa in a fine-mesh strainer and rinse under
cold running water for 2 minutes. Stir into the boiling water. Reduce the
heat, cover, and simmer for 20 minutes, or until the water is absorbed
and the quinoa is tender. Uncover and set aside. Bring a large pot of water
to a boil. Cut off and reserve the tops of the peppers. Remove the seeds
and ribs. Add the peppers and tops to the boiling water and cook for 5
minutes. Drain.

In the same pot, heat the oil over medium heat. Add the onion and
cook, stirring occasionally, for 6 minutes, or until golden brown. Stir in the
garlic. Remove 2 tablespoons of the onion mixture and set aside.

Add the spinach to the pot and cook, stirring frequently, for 5
minutes, or until wilted and any water evaporates. Remove the pot
from the heat. Add the feta, currants or raisins, almonds, and quinoa to
the spinach mixture. Stir to combine. Arrange the peppers in a shallow
baking dish. Spoon in the stuffing, mounding to fill, and replace the tops.
Add ½-inch water to the baking dish. Cover loosely with foil and bake for
40 to 45 minutes, or until the peppers are tender.

Meanwhile, in a saucepan, combine the tomatoes (with juice),
tomato paste, Italian seasoning, and the reserved 2 tablespoons onion
mixture. Bring to a boil. Reduce the heat, cover, and simmer for 30
minutes, or until thickened. Spoon the sauce onto plates and top with the
peppers.

Makes 4 servings

Per serving: 326 calories, 11 g fat (2.3 g saturated),
42.75 g carbohydrates, 9 g fiber, 14 g protein

Chicken Spinach Parm

1   Tbsp olive oil
1   boneless, skinless chicken breast
1   Tbsp Italian seasoned bread crumbs
1   tsp grated parmesan
Salt and pepper to taste
1   small clove garlic, crushed
¼   cup marinara
3   handfuls baby spinach leaves

Heat the oil in a nonstick skillet over medium heat. As the oil is heating,
pound the chicken to ¼-inch thickness, then sprinkle with bread crumbs,
cheese, salt, and pepper, pressing so the crumbs stick. Place in the
pan with the garlic and saute for 2 to 3 minutes per side. Top with hot
marinara. Add the spinach, turning frequently with tongs until it wilts.

Makes 1 serving

Per serving: 366 calories, 17 g fat (3 g saturated), 21.25 g carbohydrates,
4 g fiber, 32 g protein

The Snackin' Section

 The suggestions below work great as anytime snacks or use them as dinner appetizers. You'll love 'em.

Veggies and Pesto

What You'll Need: Pesto sauce, eggplant, tomato, peppers

With these skewers, the more vegetables the merrier! Simply grill a colorful array of vegetables topped with a light seasoning of pesto sauce. Grill until charred and then devour.

Kale Chips

What You'll Need: fresh kale, olive oil, salt, pepper

Remove stems and ribs from fresh, clean kale and then tear into large, chip-size pieces. Toss on a baking sheet with olive oil, salt, and pepper. Bake for 5 minutes at 375° F.

Tomato Bruschetta

What You'll Need: Tomatoes, garlic, basil, salt, pepper, balsamic, toast

Simply chop up tomatoes—try to remove as many seeds and juice as possible so the toppings aren't too wet—throw in some finely minced garlic, basil, salt and pepper, and a touch of balsamic. Refrigerate while you toast and break apart bite-size pieces of fiber-rich bread. Then top each golden bread-bite with the toppings.

WHAT'S FOR DESSERT?

Glad you asked! On the 14-Day Anti-Inflammatory Diet, may we suggest an apple? Maybe a nectarine? Whoa, whoa, whoa, you say, hold on there.

No dessert?

Of course not. You can have dessert on the plan, but let's remember what usually defines "dessert" in our culture. Ice cream. Pie. Leftover birthday cake. Cookies and milk. Under normal life circumstances, these are fine choices in moderation on rare occasions. However, during this two-week period, you're looking to establish much healthier eating habits, lose weight, and conquer inflammation. What do those desserts have in common? Lots of added sugar and refined carbs. Some may still have trans fats. Heck, they may even be fried (deep-fried Oreos, anyone?).

So let's have some perspective on dessert. Fresh fruit. Maybe a dollop of yogurt with a drizzle of honey. These will help you on your journey, not undo the healthy choices you made all day long. So for two weeks: Avoid added sugar, processed products, baked goods, engineered decadence, and basically anything sweet that comes with a label in the supermarket.

After two weeks of fresh, healthy eating, you may feel so good you may never want to go back to the old ways...

Food Isn't *Just* About Eating

Smart ways to use food to de-stress, calm inflammation, and lose more weight

WE'VE TOLD YOU what foods to try. Now we'll tell you how to make everything else surrounding food—the shopping, the cooking, the serving, and yes, the eating—work harder for you. A delicious meal should do more than just nourish. All the aesthetics of food can be tapped to make the entire experience healthier for your body and soul. Shopping for healthier foods, for example, should make you feel good. That cuts your stress levels. It calms your mind. It fills you with positivity instead of toxic hormones, and even those little moments added together can contribute to a healthier outlook, a slimmer waistline, and lower inflammation levels.

The best part? All of these tips are simple and quick. You can add them to your new 14-day anti-inflammatory lifestyle with little or no effort.

MASTER YOUR MINDSET

A great place to start, and the largest section in this chapter because it's so important. Your mindset—how you'll approach choices and react to surroundings—will most likely determine all your outcomes. A healthy, positive mindset leads to healthy, positive actions. It really is that simple, and that complicated. But, hey, we prefer simple, so we've assembled a host of easy-to-try tips and ideas on how to make your mindset a powerful ally.

Don't Deprive Yourself

Though you may give yourself a pat on the back for passing on that slice of chocolate cake you've been craving for dessert, you're actually doing yourself (and your waistline) a disservice in the long run. According to a study in the *International Journal of Eating Disorders*, when you resist food, your body actually experiences more cravings for whatever it is you aren't getting. Saying "no" to a sweet treat or slice of pizza wires our brains to view forbidden foods as rewards, setting us up for cravings that are hard to satisfy, so give yourself a break and indulge—but here's the key: *every now and then*. Indulge three times a day and you're sabotaging yourself.

Beware of Wedded Bliss

A review of more than 600 studies found that being married, and transitioning into marriage, are both associated with weight gain. Transitioning out of a marriage, however, is associated with weight loss. The researchers found that weight gain occurs because of increased opportunities for eating due to shared, regular meals and larger portion sizes, as well as decreased physical activity and a decline in weight maintenance for the purpose of attracting an intimate partner.

Sounds depressing, right? Let's get real. We're hardly advocating staying single or getting a divorce (unless you choose to), but this research clearly indicates that dieters need to be especially careful about post-wedding complacency when it comes to taking care of your health and weight. Our advice: You're a couple who has sworn to support one another, so do that. Shopping, meal prep, and working out can all be couple activities.

Leave Notes for Yourself

It's crucial for you to be your own driving force. Luckily, research has shown that doesn't require a tremendous amount of effort. According to a 2015 study in the *Journal of Marketing Research*, subtle, even subliminal, messages may be more effective at helping us stick to a healthy eating regimen than ongoing, conscious focus. The research showed that people who receive reinforcing notes urging them to eat healthily were more likely to make smarter choices than those who tried to keep their goals top of mind at all times, so grab some Post-Its and start crafting motivational messages!

Make a Habit of Stepping on the Scale

While having a scale in the house isn't right for everyone, research has shown that it can help encourage weight loss by providing a level of accountability. When Cornell University researchers observed dieters who weighed themselves daily, they discovered that the routine of stepping on a scale helped those people lose more weight than those who weighed themselves less frequently. To avoid being thrown off by natural fluctuations in body weight, try stepping on the scale the same time every day.

Surround Yourself with Friends

Friends are helpful not only because they can double as workout buddies or help hold you accountable for appropriate diet and exercise, but also because they're a surefire way to combat gut-growing feelings of loneliness. A study in the journal *Hormones and Behavior* found that those who feel lonely experience greater circulating levels of the appetite-stimulating hormone ghrelin after they eat, causing them to feel hungrier sooner. Over time, folks who are perennially lonely simply take in more calories than those with stronger social support networks, so be sure to fit time with pals into your busy schedule.

...But Pick the Right Dining Partners

It's always great to catch up with old pals or join your co-workers for a celebratory happy hour, but if you're watching your weight it's important to take note of who you choose to break bread with. According to an Eastern Illinois University study, you're in danger of consuming 65 percent more calories if you're eating with someone who gets seconds. In other words, while the old friend visiting from health-conscious LA may make a great dining partner, you should take a break from the co-workers who keep ordering rounds of drinks and nachos.

FOOD ISN'T *JUST ABOUT EATING*

LOL

Laughter may not be the best medicine for everything, but if you're trying to slim down, feel free to let out a chuckle or two. According to a study published in the *International Journal of Obesity*, laughing can increase your basal energy expenditure and resting heart rate by up to 20 percent, so go ahead and pull up an amusing YouTube video.

Beware of Boredom

Boredom isn't just bad for your brain, it's also bad for your waistline. According to the *Journal of Health Psychology*, boredom strips you of your ability to make smart food choices. In the end, you become an "emotional eater." What's more, boredom can turn you into the worst kind of emotional eater because you not only make the wrong food choices but also eat much more fattening foods than you normally would. To stave off boredom, *engage*. Reach out to friends, take a walk, read a book. Loitering in your own home—especially around the kitchen—is a bad look.

Dress Up For Your Meals

Nothing beats breakfast in your PJs, but you can keep your goals front and center by dressing up before a meal. Showing that you care about your appearance is a great reminder to eat in a way that reflects that, whether you're throwing on business attire or a pair of jeans.

Make Fewer Decisions

Decision fatigue is real, and it could be hindering your ability to shed some pounds. A study published in *Social Science and Medicine* found those who have high levels of what's called "skill discretion"—i.e., they exercise control

157

by getting things done themselves—tended to have lower BMIs. In contrast, those who are constantly deciding on courses of action for others may eventually come down with decision fatigue and make ill-informed choices, such as ordering that piece of cheesecake for dessert.

Manage Stress

A study in the *American Journal of Epidemiology* found that dealing with work-, finance-, or relationship-related stress can pack on the pounds. When you're stuck in a hair-pulling situation, your body releases the stress hormone cortisol, which raises inflammation and signals your body to store abdominal fat. Next time you find yourself overwhelmed, pull yourself into the moment, close your eyes, take a few cleansing breaths, and say, "Okay, now what do we need to do to handle this?" It's simple, but it's also a great way to pause and hit your refresh button.

Daydream

Who knew that fantasizing about eating your favorite candy can actually result in real-life weight loss? A study found that daydreaming about eating an entire packet of the sweet stuff before indulging may cause you to eat less of it. To come to this finding, researchers asked participants to imagine eating three M&Ms versus 30. Then, they conducted a taste test where participants were able to nosh on the chocolate orbs. The results? Those who imagined eating lots of M&Ms ended up gobbling down the least.

Take Out Your iPhone

Even if you fill up on produce, lean proteins, and whole grains, according to *British Journal of Nutrition* findings, when you think about the quality of your diet, you're likely forgetting about all the unhealthy food that also finds its way to your mouth. People tend to exaggerate the good foods they eat and underestimate the bad stuff, says study author, Kentaro Murakami, PhD of Japan's University of Shiga Prefecture. While it's not necessarily intentional, it's likely one of the reasons why it's so hard for people to lose weight. For example, you might grab a handful of candy at a co-worker's desk or a sample at the mall and then forget about it altogether. Our advice: To get a more accurate overview of your diet, keep a detailed food journal on your phone—yes, that means you should include that food court sample, too. Whether you snap photos or keep a written log is totally up to you—both tactics will work. The more food records dieters kept over the course of 30 months, the more weight they lost, a study in the *American Journal of Preventive Medicine* found.

Stop the Shame Game

In her book *The Naughty Diet*, author Melissa Milne— whose essay, "I Eat Slim-Shamers for Breakfast" also went viral—interviewed thousands of women about the body shaming, and they all said the same thing: "They were sick and tired of feeling bad while trying to be good," she writes in *The Naughty Diet*. "And here's the secret of all secrets: You don't feel bad about yourself when you get fat. You get fat when you feel bad about yourself." This could be because chronic stress raises inflammation levels, which can trigger belly fat storage. Be kinder to yourself, which will reduce stress and help you maintain a positive perspective.

Snuggle up with Your Sweetie

Not like you needed another reason to fall in love, snuggle up with your sweetie, kiss, or get it on. Harvard Medical School researchers found that all of those things can aid weight loss. How? Lovey-dovey feelings cause levels of the hormone oxytocin to increase, which in turn, decreases appetite.

Dine with a Dude

Want to stay on track with your diet while dining out? Leave your lady at home, guys. Strange but true: When men dine with women, they eat up to 93 percent more, according to researchers at Cornell University. "These findings suggest that men tend to overeat to show off," lead author of the study, Kevin Kniffin, explained. "Instead of a feat of strength, it's a feat of eating." Women, on the other hand, ate the same amount food no matter who they broke bread with. (Okay, we're not really suggesting men stop dining with women. But gents, keep this research in mind when you're eyeing your portion sizes).

Tap into Your Emotions

In a 2015 Orlando Health survey of more than a thousand respondents, the majority cited their inability to stay consistent with a diet or exercise plan as their primary barrier to weight loss success. Sounds common, but here's the kicker: Only one in 10 of the survey respondents noted their psychological well-being as part of the equation—and it's likely why nearly two out of three people who lost five percent of their total weight ended up gaining it all back. Yikes! To unlock the door to weight loss success and stop emotional eating, try keeping a journal that tracks your food choices and—here's the important part—current mood. Then, look for unhealthy patterns, which can help you recognize specific emotional connections you have with food. Once you're more aware of these connections, it will be easier to adopt healthier eating patterns. Do you always reach for something sugary when you're stressed or devour fries when you're sad? Instead, try more productive ways to cope, like going for a brisk walk or texting a friend.

Beware of Health Halos

Do you consider products from specialty supermarkets to be healthier than those from other grocery stores? Or do you think that dishes from organic restaurants are all waistline-friendly? If you answered yes to either of these questions, you could be derailing your weight-loss efforts. When people guess the number of calories in a sandwich coming from a "healthy" restaurant, they estimate that it has, on average, 35 percent fewer calories than they do when it comes from an "unhealthy" restaurant, according to a study in the *Journal of Consumer Research*. Remember that the next time you reach for that package of Whole Foods' Organic Fruit & Nut Granola. One cup of this seemingly healthy snack contains almost 500 calories. Wow.

Build a Better Kitchen

Don't worry, you don't have to rip out your cabinets and tile the floor. But your kitchen is ground zero for all your meals —as well as all the choices that shape those meals. It makes sense to take some small yet simple steps to make this environment conducive to your success. Mindset is part of this as well—your surroundings affect your mood. A happy kitchen leads to healthy eaters.

Healthify Your Kitchen

Though you may think that strong willpower is a necessary trait to overcome down-time grazing, your success is more dependent on your food environment than anything else. Most people don't have the urge to eat celery sticks; cookies, however, are different. You can't eat what's not there, so make sure when you open the pantry, you aren't tempted with the sugary, salty, fatty, inflammatory foods that most people choose when eating just to eat. Instead, stock your refrigerator with fresh vegetable slices and whole foods that will be easier to pass on if you're not really hungry.

Buy a Fruit Bowl

You know that hitting the recommended five to nine daily servings of fruits and veggies can make it easier to slim down, but that doesn't make it any easier to accomplish. A simple way to make it happen? Buy a fruit bowl. You're more likely to grab fruits and veggies over less-healthy options if they're ready to eat and in plain sight. Also, keep washed and prepared veggies like cucumbers, peppers, sugar snap peas, and carrots in the front of the fridge so they aren't overlooked. Bananas, apples, pears, and oranges fare well as sweet snacks and should be kept on the counter where everyone can see them. And don't underestimate how a colorful selection in the bowl can also lift your mood just by looking at it.

Stop and Smell that Fruit

Oh, and that fruit bowl can do more than just add ambiance. As it turns out, studies have shown that taking a whiff of fresh green apples, bananas, and pears can help curb appetite and lessen cravings for sugary desserts.

Color Coordinate

Turns out that plate color matters. Per a recent study from Cornell University, diners serve themselves more food if the color of their food matches the color of their plate. In other words, if you're eating from a white plate, you're more likely to help yourself to more rice or pasta. Conversely, if your goal is to eat less, select plates that have high contrast with what you plan to serve for dinner.

Go Blue

In addition to coordinating with your dishes, the hues you surround yourself with while you chow down can impact your appetite. According to several studies, blue is an appetite suppressant. Scientists suspect this is because there aren't many naturally-occurring blue-hued foods aside from blueberries and a handful of others. This behavior might also stem from our ancestors, who when foraging for food, stayed away from sources that were blue, black, and purple because they were believed to be poisonous. So buy some blue dishes, or freshen up your eating area with a blue tablecloth or placemats.

Hang a Mirror in Your Kitchen

In a 2015 study in the *Journal of the Association for Consumer Research*, scientists instructed subjects to choose either a fruit salad or a chocolate cake, then eat and evaluate their snack. Those who ate the chocolate cake in the room with the mirror found it less appealing than those who didn't have a looking glass nearby, but those who opted for the fruit salad reported no difference in taste. In other words, the presence of a mirror makes unhealthy foods less appealing. So hang one in your kitchen.

Proper Prep Prevents Poor Performance

Put your free time during the weekends to good use. Prepping healthy, homemade meals and snacks can help you grab a quick meal without resorting to packaged convenience foods or drive-thru quickies that are full of inflammatory ingredients.

Rethink Variety

When many of us have too many options to choose from, we often become flustered and make the wrong decision. Same goes for food. If you have a few different boxes of cereal and a handful of flavors of potato chips, you're likely to eat more of the packaged stuff. Limiting your options to just one can cut down on your grazing habits and prevent a snack attack. Overeating a big variety of vegetables, on the other hand, isn't going to hurt you. If that's your weakness, buy veggies and turn it into a strength.

Hide Your Vices

Out of sight, out of mouth? Simply reorganizing your pantry staples could translate into serious calorie savings. A study published in the *Journal of Marketing* found that people are more likely to overeat small treats from transparent packages than from opaque ones. For this reason, many nutritionists suggest keeping indulgent foods in the pantry on a high shelf so that you're less apt to mindlessly grab them.

Try Smaller Plates

The bigger your plate, the bigger your meal. How so? While smaller plates make food servings appear significantly larger, larger plates make food appear smaller—which can lead to overeating. In one study, campers who were given larger bowls served themselves and consumed 16 percent more cereal than those given smaller bowls. Swapping dinner for salad plates will help you eat more reasonable portions. To kick even more calories to the curb, use small red plates. Although the vibrant hue may not match your dining room decor, the color can help you eat less, according to a study published in the journal *Appetite*. Researchers suggest that the color red reduces the amount we're likely to eat by subtly instructing the mind to stop noshing.

Be Boring

Repetition builds rhythm. If you get into a rhythm with a few terrific and healthy go-to breakfasts and snacks, you're choices become easier. Make an effort to pinpoint these for yourself. "Hmm, I'm starving what should I have?" doesn't often end well. You can change the rotation every few weeks, but pre-set meals or workouts on certain days— while potentially boring—will help tremendously.

LOOK FORWARD TO SHOPPING

Hitting the grocery store should feel like an exercise in optimism, a chance to build excitement and positivity toward what you're trying to accomplish. Stores have more healthy choices than ever—and if you know your store, you know where the unhealthy foods are. Think of it this way: Every positive choice you make starts here. You know your mind is right when you leave the grocery store with full bags and a healthy smile on your face.

Don't Shop on an Empty Stomach

You've heard it before, but boy is it true. Grocery shopping on an empty stomach is never a good idea because research has shown it inhibits your ability to make smart choices. In a study published in *JAMA Internal Medicine*, researchers found that even short-term fasts before shopping can lead people to make more unhealthy food choices, picking a higher quantity of high-calorie foods. Do yourself a solid: Have a healthy meal or snack before you go.

Beware of Big Box Stores

Costco or Sam's Club are convenient and great money-savers, but keep the following in mind: A 2015 study in the journal *Appetite* found that the larger the bottle, bag, or box the food comes in, the larger we think the serving size should be. To come to that conclusion, researchers surveyed more than 13,000 people and found that when confronted with larger packages of sodas, chips, chocolate, or lasagna, the shoppers tended to want to serve themselves larger portions. Understand you're buying bigger packages so they last longer, and *that's* why more is better.

Make a List

Think writing a grocery list before heading to the store is a waste of time? As it turns out, it may be the key to losing weight. A *Journal of Nutrition Education and Behavior* study of more than 1,300 people discovered that shoppers who regularly wrote grocery lists also purchased healthier foods and had lower BMIs than those who didn't put pen to paper before heading to the store. Researchers hypothesize that shopping lists keep us organized, which in turn helps us fend off diet-derailing impulse buys (hello, candy aisle). Before heading to the supermarket to stock up, spend a few minutes taking inventory of your kitchen, and then write a list. Be sure to organize it by category to prevent zigzagging all over the place; that ups the odds you'll walk by—and purchase—tempting treats that could derail your weight loss success.

Don't Be Fooled By Labels

Just as big-box stores can be a psychologically tricky terrain for dieters, so to can healthy-sounding labels on the food that we eat. A Cornell University study printed in the *Journal of Marketing Research* suggests people eat more of a snack that's marketed as "low fat." Participants in the study ate a whopping 28 percent more M&Ms that were labeled "low fat" than when the colorful candies didn't have the label. If a food label seems too good to be true, it probably is.

Swap Your Noodle

The average American consumes *15.5 pounds* of pasta each year—most of it the refined white stuff. What's the trouble with that? This type of noodle is almost completely void of fiber and protein, two vital nutrients for weight loss. To boost the belly-filling fiber and hunger-busting protein in your meal, opt for a bean-based noodle like Banza Chickpea Shells (2 oz., 190 calories, 8 g of fiber, 14 g of protein) or Explore Asian Black Bean Low-Carb Pasta (2 oz., 180 calories, 12 g of fiber, and 25 g of protein). Alternatively, whip up a batch of spiralized veggie noodles.

Read the Ingredient List

The numbers on the nutrition panel aren't the most important part of a food product. You need to look at the ingredient list, too. If there are ingredients you cannot pronounce or if you see anything you think may not be a natural ingredient, put the product back on the shelf.

Use Self Checkout

Is your obsession with Reese's and Pringles derailing your weight loss efforts? It might be if you're not using the self-checkout kiosks at the grocery store. Let us explain: According to a study by IHL Consulting Group, impulse purchases dipped 32.1 percent for women and 16.7 percent for men when they scanned their items and swiped their credit card on their own. Although not all impulse buys are bad for your belly, a whopping 80 percent of candy and 61 percent of salty-snack purchases are unplanned.

Take a Stroll to the Farmer's Market

The faster food gets from the farm to your plate, the higher its nutritional value, so, no matter the season, stay healthy by heading out to your neighborhood farmer's market and stock up on fresh fruits and veggies. The walk around the market is a great way to elevate your heart rate a bit, the beneficial finds can't be beat, and it just feels good to be around fresh food (especially if the market is outdoors). To make the most of your nutritionally-minded outing, keep an eye out for what's in peak season whenever you go.

Go Gardening

Why not go shopping in your own backyard? Of all the activities you can do in an effort to shed a few pounds, gardening is one of the most beneficial and relaxing options. Research conducted by the University of Utah shows that people who garden are about 11 to 16 pounds lighter than those who don't, so throw on some gardening gloves and get to planting. For added weight loss benefits, consider planting herbs such as cilantro and mint, which combat bloating and suppress your appetite, respectively.

Don't Serve Food. Let Food Serve You

Between the moment when "Food's done!" and the plate hits the kitchen table, you have an opportunity to make your meal even healthier. Here's how to serve with smarts.

Slice Away One Slice

Making your sandwich with two slices of bread is *so* last year. Aid your slim-down efforts by opting for whole-grain bread over white and preparing your sandwich "open-faced" style—the fancy name for kicking the top piece of bread to the curb. Doing so keeps about 70 to 120 calories off your plate. If losing some bread leaves your tummy rumbling, beef up your meal by munching on a cup of baby carrots or sugar snap peas. These pop-in-your-mouth veggies are loaded with fiber and water, which can help aid satiety.

Rearrange Your Plate

Most people think of their protein or meat as their meal's main event, but that doesn't have to be the case. Try this: Place flavorful vegetables front and center on lunch and dinner plates, accompanied by sides of protein and whole grains. By simply rearranging your plate priorities, you'll automatically consume fewer calories and take in more health-protective vitamins and nutrients.

Dim the Lights

Have trouble eating reasonably sized portions? Try dimming the lights and cueing up some soft music.

According to a study published in *Psychological Reports*, soft lighting and music lead noshers to eat less and enjoy their food more. That's what we call a win-win.

Make Dinner a Buffet

When you place heaping bowls of food on the table, overeating is inevitable. In fact, a study in the journal *Obesity* found that when food is served family-style, people consume 35 percent more over the course of their meal. To avoid scarfing down extra bites, keep food on the stove or counter and spoon it out onto plates from there. When going back for seconds requires leaving the table, people tend to consider their hunger levels more carefully.

WHEN THE FOOD IS IN FRONT OF YOU

Eat Mindfully

We know you love binge-watching your favorite TV series, but it's important to enjoy your meals sitting at your kitchen table—not in front of the television. Why? In addition to commercials of unhealthy food and drinks increasing our cravings, TV is so distracting that it makes it harder to realize when we're actually satiated. A study in the *American Journal of Clinical Nutrition* found that paying attention while eating can aid weight loss efforts while distracted eating can lead to a long-term increase in food consumption.

Chew on This

A study published in the *American Journal of Clinical*

Nutrition found that chewing more and eating slowly caused participants to ingest fewer calories. How so? Chewing the food more thoroughly simultaneously lowered levels of appetite-stimulating hormones and increased levels of appetite-suppressing hormones.

Store Leftovers ASAP

When you're done cooking, portion out just enough for your meal and pack the rest away. Putting your food away ASAP will not only keep it fresh for future meals but it will also deter you from mindlessly nibbling and eating more than the desired portion size. Same goes for when you're dining out: Ask for a to-go box along with your meal, that way you can pack away the leftovers and aren't tempted to overeat. When noshing on the leftovers at your next meal, you can also experiment with adding some additional fiber or protein to give the dish a nutritional boost.

Give Your Fork a Break

We've already established how chewing thoroughly can ensure you eat a meal at a leisurely pace, but there are other tricks you can use to slow down, too, like putting your fork down between bites. A study in the *Journal of the American Dietetic Association* found that slow eaters took in 66 fewer calories per meal, but compared to their fast-eating peers, they felt like they had eaten more. While 66 calories might not sound like much, cutting that amount out of every meal adds up to a weight loss of more than 20 pounds a year.

Avoid Dinner Distractions

This goes along with mindful eating: Researchers at the University of Birmingham found that diners who were distracted at meal time consumed significantly more unhealthy snack foods later in the day than those who paid close attention to their food and avoided distractions. Try keeping your phone in another room at mealtime.

Have a Midnight Snack

Even if you're trying to reduce your eating window, you shouldn't go to sleep starved. In fact, going to bed with a rumbling stomach can make it more difficult to fall asleep and subsequently leave you feeling ravenous the next day. And get this: Eating the right type of bedtime snack might even boost your metabolism and aid weight loss. The right snack can help keep blood sugar stable so the fat-burning hormone glucagon can do its job. Try pairing a natural carb with a healthy fat. Apple slices and almond butter or carrots with guacamole fit the bill.

Cleanse Your Palate

Are your portion control issues making it harder to stay on track? Stop yourself from going back for seconds by grabbing a box of mints. People often yearn for that second cookie or helping of mac and cheese because the taste of the first still lingers. To cleanse your palate, keep mints or breath strips on hand and pop them when it's time to quit noshing. Not only will this rid the alluring taste from your tongue, it will also keep your mouth busy and act as a distraction. Drinking water or tea are also helpful tactics.

SPECIAL SECTION

A Triple-Whammy Against Inflammation

YOU'VE HEARD ALL about the food. Now discover three more powerful weapons against inflammation. Use them in conjunction with healthy eating and they'll help you lower your inflammation levels and prevent disease, to be sure. But they'll also help you lose weight and maintain your ideal weight once you get there. All you have to do is read on...

The Incredible Power of Sleep

Aside from food, it's one of your biggest anti-inflammatory weapons

WE'VE TALKED A LOT about the anti-inflammatory properties of healthy food, but if you want to do your body an even bigger favor, embrace good sleep. Why? It has incredible anti-inflammatory power. So if you're already eating well, prioritizing sleep adds an extra punch to your body's inflammation levels. Not only that, quality sleep also contributes to weight loss and disease prevention.

So let's look at easy ways to get restorative sleep into your life. Your body will thank you later.

Respect the ZZZs

When it comes to sleep, an important word to remember is *respect*. Why? Sleep may be the most disrespected part of daily life for a lot of people. When we're busy and overscheduled, we wake up earlier and go to bed later. "I can get by on 5 hours," we say. "I'll make it up on the weekend." But we never do. We lay in bed staring at screens, trying to nod off with hyperactive minds we haven't allowed to calm. If we're overweight, we may snore and develop sleep apnea, which brings even worse-quality sleep. We wake up exhausted. Later in the day our fatigue gives us hormonal junk food cravings. Our normally-healthy intentions are compromised. Our stressed bodies, surprise, release stress hormones. We become a combination of listless and agitated. And we do it all again the next night. Bad mojo.

Over time, disrespected sleep patterns lead to weight gain and, yes, chronic inflammation. One study found that poor or restricted sleep—losing 25-50 percent of a normal 8 hours—raised inflammatory markers like cytokines in otherwise healthy people. Getting a satisfying 7-8 hours a night, including the deeper, restorative cycles, allows our bodies to hit refresh. And if you're making other healthy choices during the day—eating to beat inflammation, getting regular exercise—sleep unlocks all the potential from good food and positive sweat. So trust sleep. Respect sleep. You know the basics: Put your devices away, give yourself an hour to wind down, make your bedroom dark and cool. Here are some other tips to help you make sleep time the most respected time of your day...

Rise & Shine

According to researchers, late sleepers—defined as those who wake up around 10:45 a.m.—consume 248 more calories during the day, as well as half as many fruits and vegetables and twice the amount of fast food than those who set their alarm earlier. If these findings sound troubling to you night owls, try setting your alarm clock 15 minutes earlier each day, and going to bed earlier, until you're getting out of bed at a more reasonable hour.

Crack a Window

Simply blasting the air conditioner, cracking a window open, or turning down the heat during the winter may help attack belly fat while we sleep, according to a study in the journal *Diabetes*. That's because colder temperatures subtly enhance the effectiveness of our brown fat stores— fat that keeps you warm by helping you burn through the fat stored in your belly. Participants spent a few weeks sleeping in bedrooms with varying temperatures: a neutral 75 degrees, a cool 66 degrees, and a balmy 81 degrees. After four weeks of sleeping at 66 degrees, the subjects had almost doubled their volumes of brown fat. (And yes, that means that they lost belly fat.)

Don't Sleep With the TV On

Exposure to light at night doesn't just interrupt your chances of a great night's rest, it may also result in weight gain, according to a new study published in the *American Journal of Epidemiology*. As crazy as it may seem, study subjects who slept in the darkest rooms were 21 percent less likely to be obese than those sleeping in the lightest rooms. The takeaway here is a simple one: Turn off the TV and toss your nightlight.

Catch More Zzzs

Looking for the easiest possible way to lose weight? Grab your pajamas early and log some extra zzzs. According to researchers, getting eight and a half hours of shut-eye each night can drop cravings for junk food a whopping 62 percent and decrease overall appetite by 14 percent. Mayo Clinic researchers note similar findings: In their study, adults who slept an hour and 20 minutes less than the control group consumed an average of 549 additional calories daily. That's more calories than you'll find in a Big Mac.

Open the Blinds

Instead of dragging yourself to the coffee pot when your alarm goes off, open all the blinds. Studies show that people who get direct exposure to sunlight in the morning between 8 a.m. and noon reduce their risk of weight gain—regardless of how much they eat. Researchers think it's because the morning sun helps synchronize your metabolism so you burn fat more efficiently.

Avoid Artificial Light

Sunlight in the morning is good, the blue light emitted from your electronics at night is bad, and artificial light should be avoided whenever possible. In a study published in *Proceedings of the National Academy of Sciences*, researchers found that being exposed to artificial light leads to weight gain regardless of what you eat.

Work By a Window

To help combat the negative impact of artificial light, try working close to a window. Researchers have discovered that those who sit near a window tend to be healthier than those who don't. Per a study in the *Journal of Clinical Sleep Medicine*, workers near a window got 46 more minutes of sleep a night on average, which is beneficial to weight loss, while workers who weren't near a window had more sleep disturbances. Additional research has shown that those exposed to natural light during the workweek tended to be more inspired to get outside and exercise.

Skip Nap Time

Napping may be an easy way to catch up on some missed shut-eye, but dozing off in the middle of the day does nothing to aid weight loss. In fact, research has found that people burn fewer calories when they sleep during the day and log their waking hours after the sun's gone down. Researchers at the University of Colorado at Boulder studied 14 healthy adults for six days. For two days, study participants slept at night and stayed awake during the day, then they reversed their routines to mimic the schedules of night owls. When participants slept during the day, researchers found that they burned 52 to 59 fewer calories than they did while catching their zzzs in the evening—likely because the schedule messed with their circadian rhythm, the body's internal clock that plays a major role in metabolism function. If your circadian rhythm is out of whack, a separate study by University of Colorado Boulder researchers suggested spending a weekend in the wilderness to get it back on track.

Simple Ways to Exercise

Take inflammation down a notch by taking your fitness up a notch

YOU KNOW EXERCISE is good for muscles, bones, joints, as well as your heart and lungs. You probably know that it's good for your blood pressure, cholesterol, and mental health. It also happens to be a terrific anti-inflammatory: A 2017 University of California San Diego Medical School study found that as little as a 20-minute session of moderate intensity exercise (subjects walked on a treadmill) can stimulate the immune system and trigger an anti-inflammatory cellular response. So a little goes a long way.

And that's the genius of it. You simply don't have to

make a huge time investment to get exercise benefits. This isn't a fitness book, but breaking a sweat is so simple that in just these few pages you'll find more ideas than you'll ever need. That's how simple exercise is: Start moving, get breathing, raise your heart rate, then do it again tomorrow. It doesn't have to be intimidating, or a hassle, or any other thing that will make you want to avoid it. Exercise is instantly customizable and can change in a second just based on what YOU want. You can choose your own activity, your own pace, your own time, your own distance. You can do it alone or with friends. You can take a class or go solo. You can listen to music or the sounds of your surroundings. You can go indoors or out. You can wear expensive clothing or a torn t-shirt. You can set a goal or just wing it. You can compete with others or push yourself.

All you have to do is start.

WHY YOU SHOULD TRY STRENGTH TRAINING

This much we know is true: Any physical activity is good. So even if you just walk your dog every day for 20 minutes, you're doing more for your body than a lot of people are doing for theirs. But different types of exercise deliver different benefits. Strength training or resistance training is unique because directly working muscles affects your body in different ways than, say, jogging. For example:

You grow stronger. This is obvious, of course, but consider the day-to-day benefits of greater strength: Everyday

Can't think of anything to do?
Here are some one-word answers...

- Stand
- Stretch
- Breathe
- Walk
- Jog
- Sprint
- Hike
- Bike
- Swim
- Surf
- Dance
- Lift
- Push
- Pull
- Throw
- Catch
- Play
- Garden

- Weed
- Mow
- Row
- Paddle
- Pedal
- Climb
- Slide
- Swing
- Pitch
- Putt
- Bowl
- Dribble
- Shoot
- Rebound
- Skate
- Ski
- Shred
- Dust

- Vacuum
- Mop
- Hop
- Crawl
- Ride
- Hide
- Seek
- Tag
- Bend
- Twist
- Squat
- Reach
- Shop
- Drop
- Don't
- Ever
- Stop

activities become easier. You can lift, move, and even climb stairs with less effort.

Your joints are healthier and your body performs better overall.

Muscle tissue aids the body in glucose management, so if you're overweight and insulin resistant, adding muscle can help regulate your blood sugar.

You look great. Oh yeah. The buffer you get, the better you look.

Oh, and strength training helps reduce inflammation in the body (you knew we were getting to that eventually, right?). And this works at any age: A 2015 study in *AGE Journal* studied 65 women, age 60 and older, who had not exercised in the previous six months. Researchers put them into two groups, one participating in a single phase, 8-week strength training program, and the other in a 3-phase, 24-week program that was more advanced. In the end, both groups saw gains in strength, obviously, but also significant reduction in c-reactive protein inflammation—23 percent in the novice group, 55 percent for the advanced. Another study in *Medicine and Science in Sports and Exercise* showed similar results. A group of 102 sedentary people was broken out into aerobic training, strength training, and control groups. Both exercise groups saw their CRP levels drop, but the strength training group's numbers (32 percent) dropped twice the amount as the aerobic group (16 percent).

So why not give strength training a try?

Here's a program that's simple, virtually free (you bought the book, after all), and requires a few square feet and nothing but your bodyweight.

It's called **3-3-3...**

3 EXERCISES. Pick from the suggestions in this chapter or swap in your own.

3 MINUTES. Perform each exercise for one minute.

3 TIMES. Complete the 3-exercise circuit 3 times.
(We recommend you do this workout at least three times a week, leaving a day in between to do some cardiovascular exercise like brisk walking or biking.)

It's that easy. The total amount of exercise per strength-training session is nine minutes, but you can go at your own pace. If you can't do a full minute of each exercise, that's fine. Work to your fitness level (you'll get better!). Need extra rest between minutes? Take it. The idea here is to challenge your muscles, not set world records.

Exercise Suggestions

These ideas are here for three reasons: They're generally well-known (no exotic moves to learn), hit multiple muscle groups in your body in a short time, and require no equipment and little space. You'll find many of these target some of the largest muscles/muscle groups in your body: glutes, quads, hip flexors, core.

Jumping Jacks

Stand with your feet together and your hands at your

sides. Simultaneously raise your extended arms above your head and jump up just enough to spread your feet out wide. Without pausing, quickly reverse the movement and repeat. Keep your ankles locked by pulling your toes up, and bounce on the balls of your feet.

Multidirectional Hop

Stand with your knees slightly bent. Jump forward 12 inches and land on your right foot. Hop backward to the start, landing on both feet. Repeat on your left foot. Next, do the sequence going sideways. Continue through the allotted time.

Plank

Assume a push-up position but with your weight on your forearms. Brace your abs, clench your glutes, and keep your body straight from head to heel. Hold for the allotted time.

BONUS CHALLENGE:
SINGLE-LEG, SINGLE-ARM PLANK

Assume a pushup position but with your weight on your forearms. Brace your abs, clench your glutes, and keep your body straight from head to heel. Raise your right leg and hold it for five seconds. Then lower it and raise your left leg for five seconds. Alternate legs for the allotted time.

Bodyweight Split Jump

Place your hands on your hips and assume a staggered stance, left leg forward. Slowly lower your body as far as you can, and then jump with enough force to propel both feet off the floor. Switch legs in midair and land with your right leg forward. That's one rep. Switch leg positions with each jump.

Forward Lunge

Stand with your feet hip-width apart. Step forward with your right leg and lower your body until the top of your right thigh is parallel to the floor and your left knee comes close to the floor. Pause, then return to the starting position. Alternate legs for the allotted time.

BONUS CHALLENGE:
COMPASS LUNGE

Stand with your feet hip-width apart. Step forward (or "north") with your right leg and lower your body until the top of your right thigh is parallel to the floor and your left knee comes close to the floor. Push back to standing and repeat the exercise while hitting points on the compass (northeast, east, etc.). NOTE: Northern lunges are forward, southern are reverse, east and west are side lunges. When you hit "due south," switch legs and continue until you reach north again. Do as much as you can in the allotted time.

Reverse Lunge with Rotation

Stand with your feet shoulder-width apart. Step back with your left foot and lower your body into a lunge as you rotate your upper body to the right. Return to the starting position. That's one rep. Alternate legs and rotation for allotted time.

Push-Up

Get down on all fours, placing your hands slightly wider than your shoulders. Straighten your arms and legs. Lower your body until your chest nearly touches the floor. Pause, and push yourself back up. Repeat for the allotted time.

Burpee

Stand with your feet shoulder-width apart. Squat as deeply as you can and place your hands on the floor. Kick back into a push-up position. Bring your legs back to a squat and jump up. Land and repeat.

Hip Raise

Lie face-up on the floor with your knees bent and your feet flat on the floor. Raise your hips so your body forms a straight line from your shoulders to your knees. Clench your glutes as you reach the top of the movement. Pause, and then lower your body back to the starting position.

BONUS CHALLENGE:
SINGLE-LEG HIP RAISE

Lie on your back with your right foot flat and your left leg raised so it's in line with your right thigh. Push your hips up, keeping your left leg elevated. Pause and slowly return to the starting position. Switch legs halfway through the allotted time.

Mountain Climber

Assume a push-up position. Your body should form a straight line from your head to your ankles. Without allowing your lower-back posture to change, lift your left foot off the floor and move your left knee toward your chest. Return to the starting position, and repeat with your right leg. Alternate the move with each leg quickly.

Air Squat

Stand with your hands on the back of your head and your feet shoulder-width apart. Lower your body until your thighs are parallel to the floor. Pause, then return to the starting position. Repeat for the allotted time.

Bulgarian Split Squat

Stand in a staggered stance, your left foot in front of your right two to three feet apart. Place just the instep of your back foot on a bench or chair. Pull your shoulders back and brace your core. Lower your body as deeply as you can, keeping your back foot on the bench. Keep your shoulders back and chest up through the movement. Pause, then return to the starting position. Halfway through the prescribed time, switch feet.

MORE EXERCISE IDEAS

No matter what activity you enjoy, there's always room for inspiration. Try these ideas, have fun, and keep moving...

Schedule a Workout Date

A recent *JAMA Internal Medicine* study of nearly 4,000 couples found that people are more likely to stick to healthy habits when they team up with a partner. Invite your honey to a Saturday morning run and then hit the showers together—knowing you have something steamy to look forward to afterward should serve as some additional motivation.

Do Some Yoga

While working out in general amps up your happiness levels, so does yoga. The practice has been around for centuries, and there's a reason for that: A 2017 study published in the journal *Frontiers in Psychology* found it only takes two minutes to start feelings its positive, mood-boosting effects. Warrior pose, here you come.

Step Outside Tomorrow Morning

Recent research published in the journal *PLOS One* found that getting direct sunlight exposure between the hours of 8 a.m. and noon reduced your risk of weight gain regardless of activity level, caloric intake, or even age. Researchers believe that the sunlight synchronizes your metabolism and undercuts your fat-storage genes.

Dress Down to Slim Down

University of Wisconsin researchers found that participants who wore jeans to work walked almost 500 more steps throughout the day than those who dressed up. As if we needed another reason to look forward to casual Fridays.

Eat Almonds Before a Workout

Before heading to the gym, don't forget to reach for a handful of almonds. A study printed in *The Journal of the International Society of Sports Nutrition* found that these subtly sweet nuts are rich in the amino acid L-arginine, which can help you burn more fat and carbs during workouts.

Take the Stairs

Boarding the elevator may be a mindless act, but taking the stairs instead could actually work wonders for your waistline. According to a University of New Mexico Health Sciences Center study, a person who weighs 150 pounds could lose about six pounds per year just by climbing up two flights of stairs daily.

Sneak in a Workout Before Work

According to a Japanese study, the timing of your workout may play a significant role in weight loss. The study found that when you exercise before breakfast, your body can metabolize about 280 more calories throughout the day compared to doing the same workout in the evening.

Drink 64 Ounces a Day

Water may just be the best pre-workout supplement when you're looking to shed weight. Studies have shown that strength training while in a dehydrated state can boost levels of stress hormones that hinder muscle gains by up to 16 percent. Try for at least eight 8-ounce glasses of water each day and at least 8 ounces during your workout.

Experiment with a Standing Desk

If you work at a job that requires you to be chained to your desk all day, try switching things up and giving a trendy standing desk a shot. Simply standing while you toil away as opposed to sitting has been shown to contribute to weight loss. *Bloomberg* reports that researchers at the Mayo Clinic found that standing burns about 54 calories over a six-hour day, and although that might not sound like much, those calories accumulate quickly. At that rate, you can burn over 1,000 calories a month just by staying on your feet.

Try Varied Cardio

People tend to find one workout routine and stick to it but it's important to switch things up every now and then, especially in terms of cardio. Instead of simply running or walking, try to vary your speeds as you go. Researchers at Ohio State University found that walking at varying speeds can burn up to 20 percent more calories compared to maintaining a steady pace, so get moving.

Take Part in an Outdoor Workout

Leaving the comforts of your gym can be difficult, but outdoor workouts have their own unique set of benefits. Research has shown that breaking a sweat outdoors may be more beneficial than burning calories inside. According to a study published in *Environmental Science and Technology*, exercising in a natural environment outdoors may improve energy levels and decrease stress more than working out indoors can.

Let Your Family Motivate You

Believe it or not, weight loss isn't just about exercising and eating right; research suggests what motivates you to get in shape can play a role in your success. A 2014 study in the journal *Body Image* looked at 321 college-age women and found that long-term, those who exercised primarily for appearance reasons had a harder time sticking to their fitness plans than those who worked out to maintain their health. In other words, stop envying those fit models on Instagram and instead remember that you and your loved ones are the people who really benefit when you slim down.

Blast Belly Fat with High-Intensity Interval Training

High-intensity interval training (HIIT) is a great belly-blasting option for those who already feel comfortable in the gym because it helps you drop fatty tissue and build muscle simultaneously. High-intensity interval training is when you perform an exercise at or close to your maximum ability for a short period of time and then take a brief respite and do it again (for example, you can try a 2:1 interval, meaning if you did an exercise for one minute, you rest for 30 seconds and then repeat). Any kind of exercise will do.

Muscle Up

More reason to strength train: Even when you're at rest, your body is constantly burning calories, and the "resting metabolic rate" is much higher in people with more muscle. That's because every pound of muscle uses about six calories a day just to sustain itself. If you can pack on just five pounds of muscle and sustain it, you'll burn the caloric equivalent of three pounds of fat over the course of a year, and be even closer to obtaining that lean physique you've always wanted.

Move for Two Minutes

However, if a HIIT workout or piling on muscle mass seems too daunting, simply move for two minutes. Why, you ask? Research in the journal *Physiological Reports* showed that people who did five 30-second bursts of max-effort cycling, followed by four minutes of rest, burned 200 extra calories that day. If you incorporate this technique into your workout routine just a few times per month, you can burn thousands of additional calories per year.

10-C

Cool, Calm, and Healthy

It's no wonder that chronic stress is linked to chronic inflammation. Learn how to find strength and calm...

ONE OF THE most interesting things I've ever heard about stress came during an interview with Dr. Mehmet Oz. He told me in so many words that stress isn't a *thing*, like a tumor, or a blood clot, or a virus. It's simply your body's reaction to *your* reaction. That's it. Something stresses you out, you perceive it as stress, so your body triggers the fight or flight reaction, blood pressure rises, stress hormones flood your system, and well, you know how that feels. If you're able to change your perception of things not going your way, or life pressures, or anything that stresses you out, you can change how your body reacts to your reaction.

That's important. Why? Well, as you might have guessed, research has found solid links between chronic stress and chronic inflammation. A 2017 review in *Frontiers of Human Neuroscience* looked at previous research examining the stress-inflammation link. Your reaction to stress may indeed trigger an inflammatory response from your immune system.

No coincidence, then, that the same diseases linked to chronic stress are also brought on by chronic inflammation: The most common stress-related diseases are cardiovascular diseases (hypertension and atherosclerosis), metabolic diseases (diabetes and non-alcoholic fatty liver disease), psychological and neurodegenerative disorders (depression, Alzheimer's disease, and Parkinson's disease), and, last but certainly not least, cancer.

There's more, especially about how stress can sabotage your weight loss efforts. In a four-year study whose findings were published in the journal *Obesity,* researchers measured the cortisol levels (you remember: cortisol is the "stress hormone") contained in the locks of hair they'd plucked from 2,527 men and women. They also tracked the subjects' weight, body mass index, and waist circumference. Ultimately, they discovered a direct correlation between chronic stress and *all three* of those obesity-related factors. See how everything—stress, inflammation, weight gain—all ties together?

Another study published in 2016 in the journal *Current Opinion in Behavioral Sciences* made an equally stunning case for a straight-line connection between your metabolism and your body's stress response. "Chronic stress can lead to dietary over-consumption, increased visceral adiposity, and weight gain," the researchers, from the Institute of

Neuroscience and Physiology at Sahlgrenska Academy at the University of Gothenburg, in Sweden, write in the report.

So let's dig into the third non-food weapon you can use against inflammation: a more positive response to stressors. Here are a host of ideas, big and small, that you can adopt today. Like the man said, it's all about perception...

Meditate, Meditate, Meditate

How many times do you have to learn about the merits of meditation? Chilling out has a direct impact on stress. Research out of Georgetown University Medical Center finds that after an eight-week course in mindful meditation, people with anxiety disorders lowered inflammatory markers and stress hormones in their blood by 15 percent. Meanwhile, according to a 2014 study published in *JAMA*, the simple act of sitting, focusing on your breath, and letting the world around you fade away can decrease stress, anxiety, and depression, making you feel more joyful.

You don't need to be solo in a studio with your legs crossed to meditate (though that certainly works). Meditation is about being present, focusing on your breath, and calming the mind by allowing thoughts to pass without judgment. Can't do that on your own? No biggie. Download an app like Calm or Headspace, which will walk you through guided stress busters, work to improve your breathing and, in turn, bring your cortisol levels back to normal.

Sit Up Straight

Research published in the journal *Health Psychology* finds that—compared to a hunched over position—sitting upright in the face of stress can boost self-esteem, fending off further angst. The idea boils down to something called embodied cognition, an idea that our bodies impact our emotions (and vice versa). And it could be that simply feeling taller boosts confidence, shooing stress away, researchers say. So plant both feet on the ground, look straight ahead, straighten your back while sitting tall, and feel your shoulder blades pull back and down.

Breathe the Right Way

There's a reason docs sometimes prescribe breathing exercises to people struggling with truly stressful times. Deep breathing—which encourages the full exchange of oxygen in the body—activates your body's calming parasympathetic response, lowering levels of inflammatory compounds linked to stress.

Most of us breathe all wrong. Take a deep breath. If your shoulders rise on your inhale, it's time to reassess. Try again. This time, on the inhale, push your belly out. When you exhale, contract in. Your belly should rise when you breathe in and shrink when you breathe out. Take a few deep breaths with a hand on your stomach to make sure you're doing it right.

Seek Out Nature (and Sunshine)

There's nothing a little sunshine can't fix, right? A 2015 study in *Landscape and Urban Planning* found that even just a quick walk in nature can make you feel happier. But, that's not all: Researchers also saw other benefits to spending time in the Great Outdoors, too, like decreased anxiety and better memory. It's not just the walking either: People strolling urban settings filled with traffic instead of trees didn't reap the benefits. Our bodies were designed to be in and near green spaces, forests, or the ocean, researchers say. Thus, studies confirm that these spaces are inherently relaxing. Can't get outside? Some research suggests that even looking at photos of nature can calm stressed minds (hello, new desktop background). Meanwhile, here's some more outdoor food for thought:

Head to the Park. There's nothing a quick trip to your local park can't fix. A 90-minute walk in the park can calm the mind, lowering activity in a brain region linked to depression, finds Stanford University research. A study in the *International Journal of Environmental Research and Public Health* found grabbing a blanket and a good book and hanging out in the middle of all that green space will instantly make you feel happier. In fact, the more greenery you're around, the better your mood will be. And if you don't want to head to the park, not a problem: Your backyard will do the same thing.

Go Hiking. Going on a walk around your neighborhood is one thing, but going hiking can take your happiness levels to a new high. A study published in *Ecopyschology* found that trekking through nature caused participants' stress to disappear, lowering their rates of depression and making them feel better than ever.

Say Thank You

Scientists are no strangers to the powers of gratitude. In fact, gratitude is linked to 23 percent lower levels of the stress hormone cortisol. Even more: A study out of the University of California San Diego's School of Medicine found that grateful folks were happier, slept better, had more energy, and had lower levels of inflammatory biomarkers—some of which correlated with heart health. The easiest way is to keep a gratitude journal. At the end of every day, write down three things you're thankful for. Some research finds that reflecting on the good at day's end can work to improve health (and sink stress).

Stop the Snowball Effect

Dwelling—or ruminating over things that have happened or things that may happen—is dangerous. Research published in the journal *PLOS One* finds that brooding over negative events is the number one biggest predictor of issues like depression and anxiety and plays a huge role in how much stress you experience. Instead of stewing over all of the ways life could go wrong, ask yourself: Is there anything in my control that I can change about this situation? If there are things you can change, change them; otherwise try to accept the present scenario without projecting into the future—a habit that can further a spiral of negativity.

Have Sex

Sex often comes with a chemical cocktail of hormones like "feel good" oxytocin as well as a release of endorphins. When running through the bloodstream these molecules can help us chill out. Research has shown that having sex with someone else is often linked to a drop in stress levels, when masturbation is not. One study in particular found that intercourse lowered systolic blood pressure. How's that for a prescription?

Stop *Trying* to Be Happy

Everyone wants to be happier—and likely puts loads of

effort in to achieve that goal. But a 2018 study in *Psychonomic Bulletin & Review* found that trying too hard to pursue happiness often results in not being very happy at all, usually because trying to be happy takes up all the time you could spend being happy. Instead, worry less about striving toward happiness and simply focus on being happy in the moment.

Step Away from Your Screen

Watching your favorite TV show on Netflix will obviously make you happy, but binge-watch wisely: Too much screen time does the total opposite. A 2018 study in *Emotion* found that those who spend more time playing video games, using social media, texting, and watching TV were less happy than those who had face-to-face social interaction or did activities away from the screen. So enjoy *The Bachelor*, then turn the TV off and pick up an old hobby instead.

Send Some Selfies

While too much screen time isn't good for your mental health, snapping some selfies for your friends on a regular basis can actually give your happiness a solid boost. A 2016 study published in *Psychology of Well-Being* found that using technology in this way can help you beat the blues. Plus, it's a fun way to stay connected with your best friends.

Spend Time Interacting with Others

After a long day of work, it might sound so nice to blow off your plans and spend the evening at home by yourself. The only problem with that? Social interaction is really good for your mental health. A study published in *Personality and Social Psychology Bulletin* found people experience greater happiness on the days they spend time with others opposed to spending time by themselves. So keep those plans. And perhaps focus on quality rather than quantity. One study in the journal *Developmental Psychology* found that simply being around one close friend can decrease cortisol levels, making it one of the more effective stress busters. That could be one of the reasons married people tend to have lower levels of the stress hormone cortisol.

Spend Money on Others— Not on Yourself

Buying something for yourself might feel good for a second, but the real way to be happy when it comes to spending your money? Getting something for someone else. At least that's what a 2011 study published in the *Journal of Happiness Studies* found. Plus, you'll score some serious brownie points with your friend group.

Be Kind to Others

While spending money on someone else can make you happy, being kind in general can help, too. A 2016 study in *Open Science Framework* found that simply being nice to others can benefit your well-being, whether that's opening a door for someone, dishing out compliments, or just listening to someone who needs to talk.

Practice Self-Acceptance

One thing that's sure to make you feel unhappy? Always striving to be someone else because you're not satisfied with who you are today. According to findings out of the University of Hertfordshire in England, researchers found practicing self-acceptance could make a big difference in your overall happiness, and it's the thing people practice the least. According to the study authors, that means being kind to yourself, learning from your mistakes, and giving yourself some well-deserved praise.

Spend Time with Other Happy People

When it comes to keeping your spirits up, choose who you spend your time with wisely. A study from Harvard Medical School found just one person's happiness can create a chain reaction, making everyone around them happy. And not just that: it goes beyond their group of friends to their friends' friends and their *friends'* friends' friends, and the effects can last for up to a year. That's a whole lot of people in great moods.

Spend Your Money on Experiences, Not Possessions

Having a house full of things is only going to make you so happy. According to a study from San Francisco State University, true happiness comes from buying experiences—not more stuff. So instead of spending your paycheck on a new watch, use that money to take a trip and make some memories to last a lifetime.

Plant Some Flowers

Why wait around for someone else to bring you a bouquet of flowers when you can boost your happiness levels by planting some wildflowers in your garden? A study in the journal *Evolutionary Psychology* found those blooms can boost your mood for days, so for good mental health, pick some flowers and fill up that vase on your kitchen table.

Go to a Concert

Yes, dealing with overpriced beer and unnecessary concert fees is indeed worth it. An Australian study published in the journal *Psychology of Music* found engaging with music on a regular basis—whether by dancing or by attending concerts—is associated with being happier overall. So buy a ticket and enjoy every second of the show.

Treat Your Emotional Exhaustion

Sometimes it's hard to find true happiness until you resolve the problems preventing you from being happy in the first place. A 2017 study in *Work & Stress* found that dealing with emotional exhaustion at work is one of those roadblocks. No matter what's been wearing you down at the office, getting to the bottom of the issue can totally change the way you feel.

Wear Bright, Flattering Clothes

When it comes to your happiness, your blue jeans might, well, make you feel sorta blue. A study from the University of Hertfordshire in England found the item of clothing that women wear when they're feeling sad is, more likely than anything else, jeans. On top of that, those feeling sad are also more likely to wear a baggy top. Happy clothes, on the other hand, are "well-cut, figure-enhancing, and made from bright and beautiful fabrics." Interesting, huh?

Forget about the Bad Times and Focus on the Good

There's absolutely no reason to focus on your past regrets—especially when it comes to your happiness. As a study in *Personality and Individual Differences* revealed, researchers found those who are able to see the past through rose-tinted glasses are much happier than those who focus on the negatives. So start seeing everything you've been through in a positive light, and your life will brighten up because of it.

Make a Donation to a Cause You Care About

Doing something good for others is an instant way to light up your life, and a study published in the *International Journal of Happiness and Development* took things a step further to find out what method of doing so makes people the happiest. The winner? Donors who give to a charity through a friend, relative, or social connection feel happiest compared to those who donate anonymously. You don't even have to be *really* generous. According to a study in *Nature Communications,* even being a *tiny* bit more generous can make you happier in life. That means simply being a little less selfish can give your mood a major boost.

Hang Out with Your Dog

It's nearly impossible *not* to be happy around your cute, slobbery pup, right? In a study published in the journal *Frontiers in Psychology,* researchers found simply being around your dog amps up your levels of oxytocin—one of the chemicals that makes you feel happy. So take your furry best friend for a walk, cuddle up for a movie, or play fetch; it'll lift *both* of your moods.

Rekindle Your Love of Learning

Who says you should ever stop learning new things once you've graduated from school? If there's a special interest you've developed, take a class: A 2016 study published in the journal *Arts & Health* found taking adult education classes can make you feel happier. And on top of that joy, you can also develop more self-confidence and form new relationships. Who knows—you might meet your new best friend in pottery class.

Just Say "No"

If you have too much on your plate, you need to learn to say no without regret. People who are "pleasers" tend to have difficulty declining requests because they want to be liked and don't want to disappoint others. But constantly reacting to others' needs is a recipe for added stress. Once you learn how to say no more often, learn how to delegate, especially at work. People who are perpetually stressed on the job are often perfectionists, who feel that no one can do the job as well as they can, so they try to do everything and end up performing poorly or less efficiently.

Sing Your Heart Out

It doesn't matter if it's in the shower, in the car, or in a community singing group. A 2017 study published in the journal *Medical Humanities* found that belting out some tunes on a regular basis can improve your mental health, decreasing depression and anxiety and making you feel happier overall.

Become a Plant Person

You don't need to instantly develop a green thumb, but attempting to bring some greenery into your life can do your happiness levels some good. In a 2015 study in the *Journal of Physiological Anthropology*, having plants in your space can be very soothing, helping to ease any built-up stress and lift your mood.

Do Something Creative

Who says you have to be under the age of 10 to enjoy playing with arts and crafts? Research published in the *Journal of Positive Psychology* found doing something creative every day—whether it's painting, coloring, or even making a pasta necklace—will help you flourish in life, making you feel happier and more positive.

Call Your Mom

Giving your mom some love instantly gives you a much-needed dose of love, too. In a study published in the journal *Proceedings of the Royal Society B*, researchers found something as simple as giving her a call and hearing her voice will instantly make you feel comforted, giving you that feel-good, happy feeling that will last far beyond when you hang up the phone.

Pretend You're Happy

They say you can fake it until you make it, and the same theory works with happiness. A study published in *Psychological Science* found that faking a smile when you feel stressed can actually decrease your stress levels, making you more joyful. Sure, it might feel like pulling teeth, but it can have a positive outcome.

Take a Bath

Who knew a little splash in the tub could result in so much happiness? In a study from the University of Nottingham in England, researchers found something as simple as spending time taking a long bath can amp up the joy you feel. There's nothing in the research about bubbles and rubber duckies, but they've *gotta* be worth some extra happy points.

Use a Sun Lamp

One effortless way to feel instantly happier? Just grab a sun lamp. According to the Cleveland Clinic, the ones with bright, white light can fight off depression, giving you a mood boost whenever you need it. And, the best part? They're super easy to get: Simply order one off Amazon.

Make an Effort to Meet New People

Online friends are great and all, but when it comes to your happiness, nothing beats making new BFFs face to face— at least that's what researchers found, in a 2013 study published in the journal *PLOS One*. Whether that means joining a club in your community or trying your hand at a sports league, you could make a lasting friendship that makes you all sorts of giddy.

Find Your Purpose

When you feel like you're working toward a goal in life, you feel like you have purpose. And according to the Mayo Clinic, that's one of the ways people find happiness. Figure out what excites you, what you love doing, and how you want people to remember you to figure out what your purpose is, then use that to fuel yourself and be truly joyful.

Plan a Real Vacation

And no, not one of those quick little three-day-weekend getaways. By actually using your time off and taking a real, quality vacation, you'll feel much happier—in fact, a lot of that happiness comes before you even leave. A 2010 study published in the journal *Applied Research in Quality of Life* found anticipating the trip left the vacationers beaming with joy for up to eight weeks.

Watch a Funny Video

All those hilarious cat videos making their way around the internet are actually pretty beneficial after all. A study published in the journal *Advances in Mind-Body Medicine* found those who watched a couple of humorous videos for 20 minutes had significantly lower levels of the stress hormone cortisol in their saliva than those who sat calmly and did nothing for 20 minutes, making them feel more at ease and happier overall.

Say Goodbye to Social Media

Social media has its pros, but it also has its cons. A study published in the journal *Computers in Human Behavior* found the more platforms the participants used, the higher their chances were of having depression and anxiety symptoms. While checking in on a couple platforms shouldn't be a too big of a problem, true happiness seems to come from staying a little more off the grid.

Quit Your Job and Go Solo

Quitting your job and going off on your own can seem absolutely terrifying, but it has plenty of benefits for your well-being. A study published in the journal *Work, Employment, and Society* found that out of all the different occupations out there, those who are self-employed are the happiest.

Watch Some Old Home Movies

Sometimes a little blast from the past is all it takes to up your happiness levels. A 2013 study published in the journal *Personality and Social Psychology Bulletin* found nostalgia can boost optimism, so dig out your old home movies and photo albums and prepare to be all smiles over the adorableness to come.

Light Some Vanilla-Scented Candles

The next time you decide to stock up on candles, get plenty of the vanilla options. A study published in the journal *Chemical Senses* found those who sniffed the scent were happier and more relaxed. Basically, feel free to put one in every room and light them up on the regular.

Use the Infrared Sauna

Infrared saunas—which heat your body from the inside out—can help clear up your skin and get rid of pain. Another perk, though? A 2016 study in *JAMA Psychiatry* found putting your body in those high temps can also work as an antidepressant, making you feel happy once you come out.

Bake Up Your Favorite Dessert

Sometimes the one thing that makes everything better is dessert. If you're feeling down and need a pick-me-up, head to the kitchen: Researchers in a 2016 study published in the *Journal of Positive Psychology* found doing a little cooking and baking made the participants feel less stressed, more enthusiastic, and happier overall. In other words: something only fresh-out-of-the-oven cookies can do so effectively.